T0146588

The Word

Escapes Me:

Voices of Aphasia

Mona Greenfield, Ph.D., LCSW, CCC-SLP
Ellayne S. Ganzfried, M.S., CCC-SLP

BALBOA.
PRESS

A DIVISION OF HAY HOUSE

Balboa Press books may be ordered through booksellers or by contacting:

Balboa Press
A Division of Hay House
1663 Liberty Drive
Bloomington, IN 47403
www.balboapress.com
1 (877) 407-4847

Print information available on the last page.

ISBN: 978-1-5043-6710-3 (sc)
ISBN: 978-1-5043-6711-0 (hc)
ISBN: 978-1-5043-6744-8 (e)

Library of Congress Control Number: 2016916305

Balboa Press rev. date: 11/19/2016

CONTENTS

This book is dedicated to everyone who has faced adversity and felt like giving up. Trust in yourself and never lose hope. You *can* do anything!

FOREWORD

Nicole Apostolou, MS, CCC-SLP, In Collaboration with Susan Yankowitz

Aphasia is usually described as a loss of language or speechlessness, words clear and useful for doctors, clinicians, and caretakers but clearly inadequate to the complex experience of 'wordlessness.' The playwright Susan Yankowitz faced a similar problem when her friend, the theater director Joseph Chaikin, became aphasic and asked her to write a play that could communicate the inner world of a person who could no longer communicate. The irony was not lost on either of them. But when he suggested that the central character be an astronomer, she found the premise for Night Sky, the play she ultimately wrote and he directed. As she writes in her introduction:

> "I began doing research on both aphasia and
> astronomy, and discovered the amazingly
> apt metaphor upon which the play came to
> be built: the connection between
> the black holes in the universe and the dark
> matter of the brain, areas in
> which light (understanding and thought for the aphasic) is trapped,
> invisible to the observer but nevertheless
> present and struggling to reveal
> itself. Because the mind, the intelligence of the aphasic, can often be
> intact -- in Joe's case, stunningly lucid – while the route from brain to
> mouth is, day after day, a minefield or obstacle course."

As speech-language pathologists, we are always taught the clinical background, the theory, the jargon and the techniques to treat an individual. We come in with our tools of the trade and begin the often slow process of rehabilitation. We assign home practice and give advice, but often we lack the time to sit and counsel individuals about the new world they are entering. This book hopes to offer more of the insights and understanding gleaned over the years. It is filled with the stories and perspectives of clients, clinicians, caregivers and family members, their struggles and successes, and their growth as human beings with aphasia. Obviously, many aphasics would like to revoke their membership in this group they have involuntarily joined, but time and time again, we have seen them demonstrate an extraordinary spirit and resiliency to persevere through each day as they confront, accept and even embrace their changed lives.

Look at cosmos and you see:

Great spaces between stars.

Now for me, spaces between words,

holes listening, holes talking.

I search many truth I feel but cannot express.

Ideas in head but pure— *poor* words.

I am aphasia,

Anna aphasia.

You know story Alice Won—*Wonderland*

fall down black hole

not die but explore new world

Now better my open heart.

Surprise in living, everyday.

I work find shine light.

Night sky beautiful

And miss- missing, and mystery.

Wonder—

Wonder full.

I. You.

All world.

Speech less.

We hope that this book will serve as an inspiration to those who find themselves in this 'new normal.' You are not alone.

ACKNOWLEDGEMENTS

This book was inspired by many persons with aphasia, and we are grateful to all these brave individuals. In particular we would like to acknowledge Al. Al had a stroke and is a participant in Metropolitan Communication Associates (MCA), a therapeutic community founded by Dr. Mona Greenfield for individuals with neurogenic disorders. Al relentlessly wrote compelling stories about his experiences during and after his stroke. Sharing his journey helped him process what had happened and motivated him to move forward. It was Al's writing that encouraged and empowered us to create this book. Thank you to all the courageous contributors who have honored us by allowing us to intimately share in their "aphasia journey." A very special thank-you to Al for his hope and the realization of dreams that have come from his pages of stories about aphasia. Everyone who knows Al is inspired by him!

We would also like to acknowledge the support of the therapeutic community created by the hard work of individual participants in the program, as well as their families, caregivers, and the program's professionals and professionals-in-training. They have all made the aphasia program flourish with a real sense of the whole person, not simply a person with a diagnosis of aphasia who needs to relearn language and communication skills. We are grateful to all those that have taken the time to learn about aphasia and educate others. It is through those advocacy efforts that we can increase awareness of aphasia. Special thanks to The Moth and the Museum of Modern Art (MoMA) for their collaborations. We have the utmost admiration and respect for the entire aphasia community.

This book would not have been possible without the tireless support and efforts of many people. We want to specifically acknowledge several of them.

Co-Acquisition Editors:

Nicole Apostolou
Yvonne Honigsberg
Mari Timpanaro

The co-editors assisted with planning, organizing, editing, interviewing, providing creative input, helping people with aphasia to write their stories and keeping everyone on track!

Photography

Nicole Apostolou
Ira Ganzfried
Chad Ruble
Stephen Symbolik

All Things Editorial including Editing, Formatting, Research and Advising

Courtney Brodie

Editing

Stacey Cohen
Temma Ehrenfeld

Legal Advisor

Michelle Epstein

Original Art for Book Cover

Lindy Grant

CONTRIBUTOR BIOS

Aaron

Aaron had a stroke on December 29, 2011 while working out at a gym. As a result, he had severe aphasia—he was unable to understand, speak, read or write a single word. With resilience and optimism, he attends individual and group therapies and works hard every day in regaining his language abilities. Little by little, he is getting better.

Aaron is from El Salvador and owned a tea business before his stroke. Aaron met his wife through salsa dancing. With the love and support of his wife, Aaron lives a happy life with aphasia.

Al

Al had a stroke in 2010, when he was home by himself. Prior to his stroke, he worked for an airline company and did extensive traveling. Al lives with his wife, who is his caregiver. Before this stroke, Al says he was very shy, but after his stroke he became very talkative. Al participates actively in many support groups.

Amy Samelson, LMSW

Amy is an experienced LMSW practitioner with strong alliance and engagement skills that build on where the client is at in the therapeutic process. She has a strong background in individual therapy and leading groups for clients with trauma, traumatic brain injury, and co-occurring diagnoses.

Avi

Avi had a stroke in 2007, when he was 35. His aphasia affects his speaking, writing and reading. Avi loves to gather people together (disabled and their loved ones) for outdoor sports, museum-going, and other activities. He is the founder of New York Outdoor Club, and has a penchant for extreme sports, including sky-diving and scuba diving.

He is also a tireless advocate for aphasia, and speaks to many speech therapy classrooms and other audiences. He helps train EMTs and other affiliated health professionals in recognizing and working with people who have aphasia. He participates in countless activities, including acting in plays through an aphasia group, and traveling to Israel and the Caribbean. He hopes to go back to medical school and become a doctor, specializing in emergency medicine.

Carly
Carly had a stroke in 2010. Prior to his stroke, Carly worked as an architect and was an avid skier and golfer. He traveled extensively around the world and shares his experiences with clinicians and friends. Although Carly uses a wheelchair, he is motivated to walk with the use of a cane. He is a very hard worker and never gives up.

Carly McCollow
Carly is a teaching artist in New York City. She has taught theater with the Brooklyn Academy of Music (BAM), Ping Chong & Company, Arts for All, and Theater Mitu. Carly facilitated storytelling workshops as a Lead Coach with The Moth. She has also taught Photovoice digital photography workshops with older adults through the Healing Arts Initiative. Carly is pursuing an MSW at the Silberman School of Social Work at Hunter College and has completed the Community Word Project's Teaching Artist Training and Internship Program.

Chad
Chad is the founder of Tapgram, an assistive messaging platform that he originally designed to make digital communication easier with his mother, a stroke survivor. Tapgram currently helps thousands of people stay connected with its easy-to-use interface (www.tapgram.com). Chad is a former broadcast journalist and development executive for branded entertainment, who is now a full-stack web developer. He is on the board of the National Aphasia Association. Chad lives in Brooklyn with his wife, two children, and a border terrier.

D'Angelo

D'Angelo is the father of 12-year old Nikolas, and was a studio owner, record producer, songwriter, manager, road manager and truck driver before his stroke on Easter Sunday 2011. D'Angelo has been dealing with aphasia challenges ever since. He's been working hard on speaking strategies, and has made huge improvements. Now, music is not the focus of his life. He still has his equipment, just in case he gets that musical bug back, but now he take photos, mostly of architecture, and edits the pictures. He also works out a lot. Going to the gym helps keep him focused. He always has another goal to shoot for.

Ellayne S. Ganzfried, MS, CCC-SLP

Ellayne is a speech-language pathologist and the former Executive Director of the National Aphasia Association. She is past President of the NYS Speech Language Hearing Association (NYSSLHA), Long Island Speech Language Hearing Association (LISHA) and the Council of State Association Presidents for Speech Language Pathology and Audiology (CSAP) and remains active in these associations.

Ellayne is a Fellow of the American Speech Language Hearing Association (ASHA). She was a site visitor for ASHA's Council on Academic Accreditation (CAA) and a practitioner member of the CAA for four years. Ellayne has created and managed several speech, hearing and rehabilitation programs in New York and Massachusetts. She is an adjunct instructor at Adelphi University in Garden City, NY. Ellayne has written articles and presented regionally, nationally and internationally on a variety of topics including aphasia, advocacy, rehabilitation and leadership skills.

Fran

Fran had a stroke in 1969 at age 24, due to a rare genetic blood clot factor. She continues to work hard in therapy to maintain her skills. She has a great sense of humor and an amazing smile and believes in never giving up. Fran loves individual and group therapy. She enjoys art, music and dancing. She has a home health aide, but aspires to always be as independent as possible. Her belief is to never give up.

Fred

Fred had a Traumatic Brain Injury (TBI) in 2004. He worked at the MoMA prior to his TBI. He has many interests including music, baseball and art. He enjoys therapy group activities, visits to the museums and baseball games.

Gordon Sasaki

Gordon is a visual artist based in New York City. His work explores visibility and its potential protagonist, invisibility. Towards these ideals, his art and teaching focus on diversity and inclusion.

Helen

Helen was a communication and presentation skills coach. Living with an aphasic for seven years taught her the true meaning of communication. She lives in New York City and works in real estate.

Ina

Ina is the proud goddaughter of Al, and she is eternally grateful to be a part of his life. She credits Al with making a positive impact on her life. Ina says, "He cared for me and now it's time for me to care of him."

Janet Kim

Janet Kim is a communications strategist with over a decade of experience working with organizations and individuals to express their truths and tell their stories. After working as a corporate consultant, she fell in love with good old fashioned storytelling at her very first Moth show and began volunteering for public radio and eventually teaching workshops for the Moth's community program.

Kim now leads the communications, online, and culture change team at Caring Across Generations, a national advocacy campaign working to transform our country's approach to caregiving and leveraging the power of story to support the dignity of older Americans and people with disabilities, their families and the caregiving workforce.

Janice

Jan was the co-founder and co-director of an adult basic education program for the deaf (known as the Fair Lawn Deaf Program). Ultimately, it grew to provide counseling, vocational assent, resume writing and interview practice with an interpreter. Jan is married to Charlie, who had his first stroke seven and one half years ago. He is paralyzed on his right side and has aphasia. Even with the aphasia and four strokes, Charlie has kept his pleasant and outgoing personality.

Joe

Joe had a stroke in 2009. For many years prior to his stroke, he worked for the NYC transit authority. He shares many stories about being a marine. Joe loves jazz music and cruises.

Kim Singh, MSW

Kim was an intern at Metropolitan Communication Associates (MCA) in the spring of 2014. She currently works as Deputy Director of the Department of Social Services on the island of Nevis in the Caribbean where she supervises the Seniors Division. She holds a Bachelors of Arts and a Master's degree in Social Work from Lehman College, City University of New York, and the Fordham University of New York respectively. Kim's love for social work began as the beginning of her teenage years when she had to take care of her grandmother who suffered a stroke. Although young and inexperienced to the task at hand, she reflected that she learned important lessons on respect, patience, kindness and family history.

Karen Han, MS, TSSLD, CF-SLP

Karen is a speech and language pathologist working for the New York City Department of Education. She has clinical experience working with both the adult and pediatric populations in numerous settings, such as public schools, outpatient rehabilitation, and private practice. Karen received her BS in Public Policy and Management from Carnegie Mellon University and completed her MS in Speech-Language Pathology at Adelphi University.

Larry Rosen

Larry is a senior instructor with The Moth, and manages The Moth's Community Program, which brings storytelling workshops and performance opportunities to diverse communities throughout New York and in selected cities worldwide. Larry has been teaching, directing, and producing storytelling, theater, improvisation, and sketch comedy performance for more than 20 years, through institutions including Second City and The New York International Fringe Festival.

Lee

Lee had a stroke at the age of 51. He awoke to right-sided paralysis and severe aphasia. He could read, but suddenly, he couldn't speak or write. Over time, he has made significant progress in his speaking and word retrieval, and has taken up a very active lifestyle. He loves film, tango, Japanese culture and arts, and gourmet cooking. After his stroke, he opened a French antiques gallery in Manhattan, with two partners. With his architectural background, he also bought a house with a barn in Pennsylvania, and he is renovating the barn and also building his "dream house" on the property.

Lindy

Lindy had a stroke in her 50s. She is a painter, a Buddhist, and has a loving family who is very involved with her care. She is very motivated and enthusiastically participates in all the aphasia program classes, but especially likes the art sessions. She still paints actively with her left hand, and her art is displayed on her website (www.strokebrush.com) and other exhibits around New York City. She credits her Buddhism with keeping her in a peaceful and positive state of mind.

Mari Timpanaro, LMSW, LSW

Mari is a child and family social worker currently working as a self-contained classroom paraprofessional and as the Assistant Director for Brain Balance Center of Summit. Mari worked with persons with aphasia at Metropolitan Communication Associates (MCA) as a social work intern.

Melissa DeLong, LGSW
Melissa graduated from NYU's Silver School of Social Work in 2015. During her graduate career, she provided supportive counseling to people living with aphasia at Metropolitan Communication Associates (MCA) and interned at Mt. Sinai Medical Center as a psychotherapist for individuals with severe mental illness and co-occurring disorders. Currently, she provides psychodynamic psychotherapy to adolescents and adults with anxiety and mood disorders.

Mona Greenfield, PhD, LCSW, CCC-SLP
Mona is a speech-language pathologist and clinical social worker. She has taught in many graduate programs in speech-language pathology, including NYU, and has supervised and trained students in speech-pathology and social work. She has lectured nationally and internationally. For the past 13 years, she has blended her training in speech-language pathology and social work by founding and directing the Metropolitan Communication Associates (MCA) and in her private practice.

Nicole Apostolou, MS, CCC-SLP
Nicole is a bilingually certified speech-language pathologist who has worked in both the public school and private practice settings. Her areas of expertise lie in autism with the pediatric population and neurogenic disorders with the adult population. Nicole presented at the American Speech Language and Hearing Association Convention in 2014 and has supervised and trained students in speech-language pathology at Metropolitan Communication Associates (MCA) where she currently works.

Rebecca K. (Rivky) Herman, MS, CCC-SLP
Rivky is a New York State licensed and ASHA-certified bilingual speech-language pathologist who holds a TSSLD certificate with the bilingual extension and DOH approval to provide early intervention services. She was an intern at Metropolitan Communication Associates (MCA), which inspired her to write her poem, "The Voice of Aphasia."

Rob

Rob had a stroke when he was 27 years old, and 3 strokes followed. Now he works out at his gym to keep physically fit and goes to individual and group therapy every week. He enjoys being with his wife, whom he met after his stroke. He spends time with his family, reading, and watching films—and he loves his coffee, too. Rob is independent, good-natured, and has made a lot of progress with his speech and other communication strategies.

Stephen Symbolik, MA

Stephen received both his bachelor's and master's degrees at the Catholic University of America in Washington, DC. He has also studied in Italy and completed course work for a Master in Theology at the Washington Theological Union. He has a diverse work background and has experience in teaching, training, community relations, regulatory management and accreditation, writing, and editing. He was the Program Coordinator for Aphasia Awareness Training with the National Aphasia Association in New York City. Currently, Stephen is the managing Editor of Fire Lines, the official publication of the Uniformed Firefighters Association of New York City.

Susan Bluhm, RN

Susan is a nursing professor and coordinator of the certified nursing assistant program, as well as a professor of the clinical lab specialist program at Truckee Meadows Community College (TMCC) in Reno, NV. She was a director of nursing at a county prison; director of staff education in several skilled nursing facilities; a psychiatric nurse in a psychiatric hospital and a pediatric nurse. Before she went back to nursing school, she was the Dean of a business school. She has had personal experiences with speech disorders and aphasia in her family.

Tamar

Tamar suffered a traumatic brain injury in her 60's. She was born in Russia and is trilingual with fluency in Russian, English, and Hebrew. She was a nurse and has actively participated in cognitive therapy to improve her communication skills after her stroke. Tamar also continues to work very hard to improve her English skills.

Yvonne

Yvonne contributed to this book, and took part in editing it, despite the challenges of aphasia. She volunteers for several organizations, including AmeriCorps Early Childhood Literacy Program; SHARE, a breast and ovarian cancer support organization; Center for Independence of the Disabled, New York (CIDNY); English Speaking Union (ESU) as an English conversation tutor; and as a volunteer coach for The Moth, a storytelling workshop. She is also an interviewer for *Visible Lives: Oral Histories about the Disabilities Experience*. She writes a blog called *Another Day in Paradise*, mostly about life post-stroke. Yvonne is an intrepid traveler, most recently climbing up endless, rocky, ancient steps in Pompeii, Italy—limp and all.

INTRODUCTION

The Birth of a Program for Aphasia

Mona Greenfield, PhD, LCSW, CCC-SLP

Throughout the development of this book, I have been so moved by the outpouring of stories, reactions, awareness, struggles, ultimate inner peace, and support created by this therapeutic community of individuals touched by aphasia either professionally or personally.

When participants in my program came to me wanting to share their stories about stroke and aphasia, I began to reflect and re-evaluate my program and my professional self. The development of this program, one which integrates care for individuals who have had a stroke and aphasia, evolved from input from participants, family members, and many interns and professionals who were committed to thinking about these individuals, those who had had a stroke and subsequent aphasia, in a special way – remembering that they are real people who had been functioning in the mainstream of the community. I was touched by these participants, their humanness, their desire to tell their stories and share their journey as we worked together.

It was through the integration of interns training with me, professionals working with me, individuals coming from a medically-focused facility or program, and my bend toward "wholeness" and desire to treat the total person that led to the creation of an approach that seemed to work. It made each person with aphasia feel less like a patient and more like one who was healing—one who could reenter the community with confidence and a sense of hope.

The many voices shared in this book reflect those individuals who want to discover a better way to approach the clinical diagnoses of stroke and resulting aphasia; family members and caregivers struggling with a changed loved one, interns who are trying to connect their professional training with clinical practice in helping people whose lives have been significantly changed, those with aphasia, and professionals who are learning through a holistic model to integrate the medical, speech-language and cognition, and psycho-social dynamics.

Through our program we exude genuine caring, instill courage, and believe that persons with aphasia, who have had their lives radically changed, can heal and find a new path.

It is by sharing in our participants' frustration, anxiety, fear, depression, and uncertainty about what the future will bring, as well as their courage, hope, faith, and strength to continue their life journey, though altered, that my team has learned many lessons:

1. Continue to believe that ongoing changes can happen in the healing process.
2. Listen to persons with aphasia and support their feelings and desire to be whole.
3. Find ways to maximize independence for the person with aphasia.
4. Include caregivers in the healing process and offer support and hope while helping them understand what the new normal means.
5. Celebrate present moments and acknowledge both progress and frustration.

CHAPTER 1

Let's Talk about Aphasia

Ellayne S. Ganzfried, MS, CCC-SLP

Ask ten people on the street if they know what aphasia is, and it is likely that half have never heard of it. It is also likely that those who have heard of it cannot give an accurate definition. Aphasia is an acquired communication disorder that impairs a person's ability to speak and understand others but does not affect intelligence. Most people with aphasia also experience difficulty reading and writing. Because people with aphasia can think as they always have but have lost the ability to use language to convey their thoughts and/or understand others, they often use the word "prison" to describe their condition. Imagine the frustration of knowing what you want to say but not being able to say it and/or saying things that others cannot understand.

Aphasia is experienced in 21-38% of all individuals with acute strokes (Berthier, 2005), and about 795,000 Americans each year suffer a new or recurrent stroke (strokeassociation.org), making stroke the most common cause of aphasia. Other causes include head injuries, brain tumors, migraines or other neurological conditions. Aphasia can also result from frontotemporal degeneration (FTD), corticobasal degeneration (CBD), and other neurodegenerative disorders referred to as primary progressive aphasia (PPA), which is a clinical dementia syndrome.

Aphasia knows no boundaries and can be acquired by all ages, races, genders, and cultures. It is difficult to get an accurate statistic of incidence, but most agree that there are between one and two million Americans with aphasia, or 1 in 250 people. Despite these numbers, aphasia typically is not recognized or understood, even by some health professionals, compounding its devastating consequences. Too often people with aphasia are discharged from a hospital without knowing their condition has a name or that they can improve with time, speech-language treatment, and community support. People with aphasia are at a tremendous disadvantage in today's health care system, where the ability to access resources is often closely tied to the ability to advocate for oneself.

Because it involves communication, aphasia affects almost every aspect of a person's life. In a survey done by the National Aphasia Association (NAA) in 1988, many people reported that friends and even family members stopped coming to visit, because they could not communicate with the person with aphasia (PWA).

Family members may also feel strong emotions—anxiety, anger, confusion, depression, despair—and family roles may be reversed. Marriages change, and partners may feel a sense of loss. There may be tension among family members and feelings of frustration and helplessness. The condition may seem hopeless. Children may feel neglected and may find it difficult to have a parent dependent on them. It is natural to go through a grieving process when a family member develops aphasia, and family members need to be helped through this process. According to G.A. Davis "an individual's aphasia is a family problem" (1983).

Many people with aphasia cannot continue to work at jobs that require extensive reading or speaking. Health insurance coverage for services may be limited. If a person pays privately for speech therapy or other rehabilitation services, aphasia can be financially ruinous. Many people with aphasia are prone to depression due to the feelings of social isolation that result from their communication difficulties.

People with aphasia report significantly worse health-related quality of life (QoL) than stroke survivors without aphasia, and worse QoL than healthy controls, particularly in the areas of independence, social relationships, and aspects of access to the environment (Hilari, Needle, & Harrison, 2012). While people with aphasia report prioritizing communication goals in their overall rehabilitation process, they also emphasize social, relationship, leisure, and work goals, as well as the need for information tailored to their needs (L. Worrall et al., 2011).

Communication partner training should be provided to improve the communicative environment provided by frequent communication partners for the PWA. Communication partners can be caregivers, family members, friends, volunteers, students, etc. Training can be provided in strategies to facilitate communication and education regarding aphasia, as well as counseling to deal with the psychosocial aspects.

"Communication partner training was shown to be an effective approach for improving communication activities and/or participation of some communication partners and is probably effective in improving communication activities and/or participation of some persons with chronic aphasia when they are interacting with trained communication partners" (Simmons-Mackie et al., 2010).

There are many misconceptions about aphasia, including the belief that people with aphasia are:

- psychologically ill,
- under the influence of drugs/alcohol,
- hard of hearing/deaf,
- confused,
- unwilling to try, and/or
- elderly.

We all must work hard to dispel these myths and provide accurate information about aphasia. Organizations like the NAA (aphasia.org) were created to educate the public to know that the word "aphasia" describes an impairment of the ability to communicate, not an impairment of intellect. The NAA makes people with aphasia, as well as their families, support systems, and health care professionals aware of resources to aid in recovering lost skills to the greatest extent possible, compensating for skills that will not be recovered and minimizing the psychosocial impact of the language impairment.

Aphasia can co-occur with other motor speech disorders like apraxia and dysarthria. Apraxia is a motor planning disorder in which the messages from the brain to the mouth are disrupted. Even though the muscles are not weak, individuals with this disorder cannot coordinate the muscle movements to say the intended sounds correctly. Dysarthria results from impaired movement and weakness of the muscles used for speech production. Individuals with this disorder may have slow, slurred, and/or imprecise speech. As with aphasia, the type and severity of the apraxia or dysarthria depend on the nature of the brain damage.

There are many different types of aphasia, and categorizing different subtypes can be complicated. Below are some of the most common classifications, as well as additional resources for accessing more comprehensive descriptions (Davis, 2015).

Global Aphasia – This is the most severe form of aphasia and is applied to those who can produce few recognizable words and understand little or no spoken language. Persons with global aphasia can neither read nor write. Global aphasia may often be seen immediately after the patient has suffered a stroke, and it may rapidly improve if the damage has not been too extensive. However, with greater brain damage, severe and lasting disability may result.

Broca's Aphasia – This is also referred to as expressive aphasia or non-fluent aphasia. In this form of aphasia, damage is typically in the anterior portion of the left hemisphere. Speech output is severely reduced and is limited mainly to short utterances. Content words (nouns and verbs) may be preserved but sentences are difficult to produce due to the problems with grammar, resulting in "telegraphic speech." In its more severe form, spoken utterances may be reduced to single words. The person may understand speech relatively well and be able to read, but be limited in writing. Broca's aphasia is often referred to as a "nonfluent aphasia" because of the halting and effortful quality of speech.

Wernicke's Aphasia – (This is also referred to as Receptive Aphasia or Fluent Aphasia.) Here, the damage is typically in the posterior portion of the left hemisphere. The ability to grasp the meaning of spoken words is chiefly impaired, while the ease of producing connected speech is not much affected. Reading and writing are also often severely impaired. Comprehension is poor and in many cases the person produces jargon, or nonsensical words and phrases, when attempting to speak. These utterances typically retain sentence structure but lack meaning. The person is usually unaware of how they are speaking and may continue to talk even when they should pause to allow others to speak; this is often referred to as "press of speech."

Anomic Aphasia – The most prominent difficulty in this case is in word-finding, with the person using generic fillers in utterances, such as nonspecific nouns and pronouns (e.g., "thing"), or circumlocution, where the person describes the intended word. It is like having the word on the "tip of your tongue." Comprehension and repetition of words and sentences is typically good; however, the person may not always recognize that a word they have successfully retrieved is the correct word, indicating some difficulty with word recognition. Difficulty finding words is as evident in writing as it is in speech.

Primary Progressive Aphasia – A clinical dementia syndrome in which language function slowly declines, due to progressive, neurodegenerative brain disease, eventually affecting additional cognitive, behavioral, and functional domains. This is in contrast to aphasia acquired as a result of a stroke or brain injury. Mesulam first used this term in 1982; he defined it as a "focal dementia characterized by an isolated and gradual dissolution of language function" (2001). With this type of aphasia, language deficits emerge and progress slowly. It is most prominently manifested in word-finding pauses, paraphasia, agrammatism, and difficulties with reading and comprehension. Other types of mental processes are relatively intact initially, but begin to decline with time.

Some of the characteristics of aphasia may also occur in isolation. This may be the case for disorders of reading (alexia) or disorders affecting both reading and writing (agraphia). Acalculia, or difficulty with math and numerical skills, can often accompany aphasia as well, yet in some instances patients retain excellent calculation skills in spite of the loss of language.

There are many types of aphasia and symptoms can vary greatly, but all people with aphasia have difficulty communicating. Aphasia can range from mild, in which a person is unable to name an object or retrieve a word, to severe, in which any type of communication is virtually impossible. As individuals with aphasia recover, their symptoms may change, which will also change the classification of the type of aphasia. It is best to check with a neurologist or speech-language pathologist to confirm that the correct type of aphasia has been identified. Speech-language pathologists can evaluate and recommend the type of speech therapy that would be most beneficial. It is important that the family understand that their loved one with aphasia is still the same person and has retained his or her intelligence. They need to keep the person engaged in life and in the activities they enjoy. People with aphasia can continue to improve over the years. Improvement is a process that involves helping the individual and family understand the nature of aphasia and learn new strategies to communicate.

Recommended communication strategies include the following (www.aphasia.org):

- Ensure you have the person's attention before you speak.
- Minimize or eliminate background noise if possible (sirens, TV, radio, and other people).
- Keep your own voice at a normal level.
- Keep communication simple but adult.
- Confirm that you are communicating successfully with "yes" and "no" questions.
- Repeat statements or directions when necessary.
- Give the person time to speak; resist the urge to finish sentences or offer words.
- Communicate with drawings, gestures, writing, and facial expressions.

It is often difficult to understand the day-to-day difficulties and frustrations experienced by a person with aphasia. One can get caught up in the technical jargon and forget the practical implications a communication impairment has on the person, friends, and family.

People with aphasia may find it difficult to:

- Take part in a conversation
- Talk in a group or noisy environment
- Read a book, magazine, or road sign
- Understand or tell jokes
- Follow the television or radio
- Write a letter or fill out a form
- Use the telephone
- Use numbers and money
- Say their own name or the names of their family members
- Express their immediate needs, ideas, or words
- Leave the home

Friends and family living with aphasia may find it hard to:

- Slow down
- Resist finishing sentences
- Adapt the way they communicate
- Keep the conversation going
- Understand what a person is saying
- Know what to do

Adapted from (ukconnect.org).

One needs to be sensitive to the needs of the person with aphasia and their family and friends. Professionals should find out what is important to the person with aphasia and focus intervention efforts on those areas. Social interaction and community engagement go hand-in-hand with direct therapy. Everyone is entitled to services, and services must be available as needed at all stages of aphasia. (LPAA, Chapey, Duchan, Elman, Garcia, Kagan, Lyon & Simmons-Mackie, 2000). No two people with aphasia are the same, and each person must be seen as a unique individual. It has been said that if you meet one person with aphasia then you have met one person with aphasia, because no two people are alike. There are many challenges with aphasia, but it is possible to live with it successfully.

CHAPTER 2

The New Normal: Recovery and Healing
Mona Greenfield, PhD, LCSW, CCC-SLP

The World of Aphasia

In the land of aphasia, a persistent voice echoes, "Here. Here! No! Yes," pointing to a cup. Does this mean "Want water, yes or no?" "No," says the voice. Maybe it is asking for juice or just trying to make sense of a jumble of language. Here it is challenging to get out the words. Feelings of helplessness prevail, and yet the desire to communicate and connect is still present. What happens to the *person* who has had a stroke or brain injury resulting in aphasia? As communication skills go awry, the person (s) with aphasia (PWA (s)) is/are, but is/are not, the same person. One person says, "I want to be a doctor." Another struggles with resuming her professional artwork. Yet another, who was married, lost his life partner due to his extensive care needs and a very changed personality. Stroke and brain trauma affect each person differently, but each person's sense of self is altered, resulting in a serious detour in his or her life journey.

In the world of aphasia rehabilitation, there are many therapies to help the PWAs regain skills. Although aphasia affects speech and language, PWAs who have suffered a stroke or brain trauma are also impacted in many other ways due to changes in their communication abilities. After an individual suffers an acute brain trauma and is hospitalized, assessments are made by the therapy team regarding ambulation/gait skills, gross and fine motor skills, and receptive and expressive language skills. Each professional works on the individual's treatment plan and objectives in an effort to facilitate increased skill level and independence for these patients. The PWAs are then introduced to many therapies as needed, such as physical, occupational, and speech-language therapy.

In addition to receiving different therapies, the hospitalized *person* with brain trauma and/or aphasia receives many visits from the doctor and has nurses coming in and out of the room constantly. He or she experiences a lot of confusion about what has happened, what is occurring while in the hospital, and what will happen when discharged. Many questions arise for the person: Will I be able to walk? Will I be able to speak? Will I be able to listen and understand? Will I be able to work? They may also have trouble requesting help, expressing feelings, and just participating in social activities. There are no clear answers to give to patients, except that it will take time.

Traditionally, when PWAs are discharged from the hospital or an acute care rehabilitation center, they are referred for outpatient therapy. They come for their individual therapy session on the day of their appointment for speech-language therapy, physical therapy, or occupational therapy and then leave the clinic. The therapy sessions offered will vary in frequency depending upon need and insurance eligibility and benefits. These sessions generally last about 30-45 minutes. Most facilities offer just individual sessions. There are some, however, that provide therapy groups. These groups provide the opportunity for the PWA to meet others who are experiencing similar difficulties. After therapy sessions, PWAs are oftentimes left feeling alone, isolated, and frustrated.

The rehabilitation process is slow and can be confusing. Facing the "new normal" means dealing with varying changes in how one functions. Certainly being able to communicate in the world becomes challenging.

There are also a limited number of therapeutic centers that provide the necessary range of therapy services and social activities. These few resources and health insurance constraints oftentimes restrict rehabilitation options for PWAs, and it is commonplace for them to spend many hours alone in the community.

Once health insurance is used up, clinics discharge the PWA. The medical team then informs him or her that the rehabilitation process is time-limited and most changes will take place within six months post stroke. Many PWAs tell me that they have been discharged from outpatient services, and that they feel frustrated, depressed, and not whole. They have difficulty adjusting to this "new normal."

Rehabilitation takes time and a lot of support is needed as the PWA reenters the community.

Aphasia affects speech and language, but the whole *person* ultimately is affected by the experience. The psychological and social self struggles to understand a changed path and significant revision of life goals and dreams. The rehabilitation process is a long and arduous road. Once discharged from the hospital, the person who has had a stroke or brain trauma may also be seen on an outpatient basis at the hospital, as needed, to continue working on their skills. Oftentimes these services are limited based upon the progress level of the person with aphasia and available health care insurance. Health insurance will frequently only pay for therapy with substantial documented progress, but progress takes time and is not necessarily consistent. There are days that are difficult for PWAs and progress can seem very slow.

Some patients are transferred to a rehabilitation facility following their period of hospitalization and receive therapy services there. The person with aphasia has to deal with shattered hopes and dreams and the loss of life as they knew it. At Metropolitan Communication Associates (MCA), the creation of a therapeutic community has been our solution to the feelings of lost identity and the struggles of working towards regaining skills and maintaining relationships. As much as rehabilitative therapies are important for those with aphasia, so too is the support for rebuilding self-esteem, recovering from feeling like "damaged property," and rebuilding relationships with employers, employees, relatives, and friends. And so the story begins. Rehabilitation and wholeness are the path.

The Welcome

When a person with aphasia contacts me, a new journey begins. Integrating many pieces of the person's self is the foundation of creating a plan to facilitate "rehabilitation." What does rehabilitation mean? Is it about learning to compensate for post-trauma "deficits," or is it more about how the person has changed? Is he or she more than just language or words? As the person with aphasia leaves the tangled medical system, they arrive at my practice, beginning the healing journey spiritually, physically, emotionally, socially and cognitively. While the medical system has done their part, individuals may be left feeling confused and overwhelmed about how they can resume their life. Oftentimes PWAs cannot continue their work and are confronted by many new challenges: hemiparesis, ambulatory difficulty, communication impairment varying in degree (which can include processing information), word finding, verbal difficulties, apraxia, and difficulties with reading, writing, and numeric information. Social isolation can also occur, as the individual feels that he/she cannot communicate properly in many relationships.

The healing process requires education, support, and therapy to move forward with life's challenges. The rehabilitation path involves more than a "medical fix." PWAs need to feel functional and whole, believing that they can continue moving forward. A sense of wellness is a critical piece in the rehabilitation endeavor.

As participants enter my program, they are provided with a dynamic assessment to identify strengths and weaknesses in their communication skills, in addition to endless support through counseling, different types of therapeutic and/or support groups, and engagement in a social community.

A speech-language-cognition assessment is done to identify areas of competence and areas that need improvement. Based on the analysis of the assessment, an individual speech-language program is developed. The most important step is helping the person to "accept" what has happened. Helping the person to realize that they will not return to functioning the way they did before is a slow, ongoing process. Aphasia continues changing as therapy progresses and the PWA begins to achieve success. PWAs certainly do not reach an endpoint six months after brain trauma as the medical establishment often tells them.

Research demonstrates that a person's speech can continue to improve years after reaching what may be deemed a "plateau" in skills by third party reimbursement. According to Kleim and Jones (2008), neuroscience research has begun to understand the adaptive capacity of the central nervous system (plasticity). The existing data strongly suggests that neurons, among other brain cells, possess the remarkable ability to alter their structure and function in response to a variety of internal and external stimuli, including behavioral training. They note that neural plasticity is the mechanism by which the brain encodes experience and learns new behaviors. It is also the mechanism by which the damaged brain relearns lost behavior in response to rehabilitation. The ability of the nervous system to wire and rewire itself in response to lasting changes in experience has become known as experience-dependent plasticity.

The principles of experience-dependent plasticity have implications for determining the most effective treatment intervention protocols. These include the following:

1. **Use It or Lose It** – Failure to drive specific brain functions can lead to functional degradation.
2. **Use It and Improve It** – Training that drives a specific brain function can lead to an enhancement of that function.
3. **Specificity** – The nature of the training experience dictates the nature of the plasticity.
4. **Repetition Matters** – Induction of plasticity requires sufficient repetition.
5. **Intensity Matters** – Induction of plasticity requires sufficient training intensity.
6. **Time Matters** – Different forms of plasticity occur at different times during training.
7. **Salience Matters** – The training experience must be sufficiently salient to induce plasticity.
8. **Age Matters** – Training-induced plasticity occurs more readily in younger brains.
9. **Transference** – Plasticity in response to one training experience can enhance the acquisition of similar behaviors.
10. **Interference** – Plasticity in response to one experience can interfere with the acquisition of other behaviors.

Wholeness and Wellness

Speech-language, cognitive therapy, and supportive counseling in individual and group contexts are recommended to treat the person with aphasia in a holistic way. In speech-language and cognitive therapy, skills affecting word finding, reading, writing, producing words, processing information, and producing numeric information and conversation are developed. The goal is to help the person regain skills and use compensatory strategies. For example, while attempting to state numbers for an address, date, or phone, teaching the person to count in a rote manner beginning with "one" may help. When attempting to produce a word that does not come out as expected, semantic feature analysis (SFA) may be utilized to describe the person, event, or place. Of course, conversation is most important to the participant. This is his or her doorway to the world and all social communication.

A combination of individual and group therapies helps the person to regain speech-language skills, as well as to gain confidence to engage in social contexts. At MCA, many groups are offered to provide emotional support and to reinforce the social self, including relaxation group, support group, literature group, music group, current events group, cognitive group, story group, and trivia and reminiscence group. During these groups, participants share experiences, feelings, and knowledge about the world. This group process is normalizing by helping participants feel valued and active in discussing what others who did not have brain trauma enjoy chatting about. Below is a description of these groups along with clients' personal experiences.

Relaxation group utilizes breathing techniques and creative visualization to give participants a peaceful, healing journey into their inner selves. Healing is facilitated through guided imagery, meditative music, and positive affirmations. This process promotes increased acceptance, self-love, and a way to connect the spiritual and emotional process with the rehabilitative work. In this way the group focuses on the whole person.

> *For Tamar, relaxation group helps energize her by providing tools for calming herself, which ultimately helps her stay focused. She enjoys the quiet time and inner work of feeling her body gently relax with full breath and guided imagery.*

Support group is an open and safe arena for participants to vent, obtain concrete help, new directions, and hope. Ongoing emotional and informational support is provided by participants and clinicians. As a social experience, this group helps participants integrate into the community as they share, exchange, laugh, cry, dream, hope, plan, learn, and love through the personal, as well as the social past, present, and future.

Al learned the tools of relaxation and began to apply these techniques in his daily life. Realizing that he was not alone, and that others shared similar experiences and feelings, helped him to accept what had happened to him with less fear and empowered him to control his stress level. Al had been a productive man who worked for an airline for many years. He struggled after his stroke, not only with speech and language, but with feeling inadequate as a husband and "a less than functioning" man. Al agreed that mind/body connections are extremely important in the healing process:

"During relaxation, we visualize a nice calm, quiet place, like a beach or a beautiful rain forest. One time I was so relaxed, I was bending toward the floor. It's visual meditation. In support group, we talk about anything that's on our mind—not necessarily about our disabilities. We congratulate each other, like seeking higher education, or moving to a new place. We are there to support someone facing surgery, anything life throws out at us! The hardest part is hearing someone talk about lack of family or friend's support. We are there for each other, even those who are quiet. Both groups are fun and stimulating and it makes it KNOWN that we're not ALONE."

Literature group participants read, discuss, and share their opinions and reactions to characters in a play. Poems and short stories are also used to engage participants in feeling comfortable with both reading and offering their views about the chosen literature. This process facilitates practice with processing information and expressive skills. Participants feel increased confidence and enjoy the forum to "chat" about literature in a high-functioning group activity. Ultimately, this group is both therapeutic and social.

Yvonne came to the program expressing concern about her ability to get her words out. She was self-conscious about the slow process in communicating, increased by her apraxia, which affected her skills in combining syllables to form words. She began individual therapy twice a week, including drill work and conversational practice. In order to reach her important goal to increase confidence and facilitate greater comfort in all social situations, Yvonne joined literature group. She read, conversed, and shared her insights and opinions in a structured group that promoted conversation. This strategy took into consideration her wholeness, feelings of self-worth, and ability to communicate with a range of communication partners.

Music group is an enjoyable method of targeting therapy by listening to music selections and reading about composers, singers, and musicians. It incorporates reading, processing information, recalling information, and discussing and offering feelings and opinions about a range of music. At MCA, we have three music groups, each dedicated to classical, pop, or jazz. Here participants are doing what people like to do socially, but in a communicatively supportive setting.

Fred enjoys listening and dancing to the music. He expresses when he likes or dislikes a genre and often sings along with the music played. Through this normalizing experience he interacts with others and feels empowered.

Current events group is where participants discuss world and local news, providing a comfortable and nurturing setting for discussing what is in the newspapers and on televised news and what is going on in the community. Being able to communicate in a supported manner, which may include using an iPad or white board to draw or write to express feelings, thoughts and knowledge, offers PWAs an opportunity to better communicate and integrate into the community with peers, family, and personal aides.

Joe always has comments about the news headlines we bring for the group. Even if he sleeps through relaxation group, he has lots of opinions to share in current events. Word finding is a challenge for him. As a veteran, and with a background working for the transit system, he always wants to have topics relating to these fields brought to the table. He also loves sports; whenever there are special games or Olympics, he becomes vociferous. Somehow he manages to get out his words and feels good about communicating in a "safe place." The therapy team and other participants support his communication, and he feels a sense of accomplishment and belonging to the therapeutic community. In this safe space, his views and opinions matter, and he is truly a member of the community.

Cognitive group offers interesting thematic conversations and includes reading, writing, memory/recall, and opportunities to organize information in a structured group. We always have interesting materials to help participants feel knowledgeable and empowered. Themes can include trips, recipes, famous landmarks, or movies to promote conversation, confidence, and increased independence connecting with others.

Carly is a young man who had a stroke. Prior to his stroke, he worked as an architect, traveled extensively, and enjoyed skiing and golf. As we create themes of travel, sports, and other worldly topics, he is always engaged and excited to share his experiences and practice his communication skills. He remains very determined to reach us with his ideas and viewpoints. His perseverance continues as he shares this information from cognitive group with his family. He continues to feel important, confident, and valued, facilitating a sense of healing and wholeness.

Storytelling group offers participants an opportunity to share stories generally focused around their aphasia. Each member has the chance to create a story over time within the structured and supported context offered by clinicians. Story organization is used to enhance participants' skills in relating organized information in a social setting. Potential struggles and successes are reviewed each week as each participant's story grows and becomes clearer, with a focus on sharing personal events and feelings with a group. As these stories develop and are shared with the group, this process supports the individual participant's comfort level with his or her sense of self and helps he or she to relate the stories in the larger community with family and friends.

> *Fran, a 69-year-old woman who had a stroke at age 25, felt alone, abandoned, and scared about how she would manage in the community. Fran shares many stories from life prior to her stroke and her long rehabilitation process. She remains proud of this journey and her goal of remaining independent. The laughter and joy from being able to relate her stories helps with feeling connected to other people and offers an opportunity to practice narrative communication skills. Engaging in a storytelling process means feeling more whole and connected to others. In this way Fran feels more positive about herself.*

Trivia group participants discuss information and facts about specific themes in a game format. Members enjoy recalling events from the past and present in categories such as music, art, and film. Through this exchange, participants feel more comfortable engaging in discussions in a social manner.

> *Fred, a 44-year-old man who suffered a traumatic brain injury, feels proud when he responds accurately to trivia questions about music throughout the decades from 1970-2010. He enjoys the challenge of recalling information and feeling connected to the world of politics, music, TV shows and a myriad of other themes used in trivia group.*

Reminiscence group facilitates remembrances of earlier decades or themes relating to personal, earlier life experiences, such as favorite childhood games, historic events, and family memories. Most of these themes are connected to life before aphasia. Allowing for and supporting this discussion helps participants piece together their personal stories, experiences, and feelings and integrate their senses of self before with their current lives with aphasia.

> *Lee enthusiastically shares information during reminiscence group. He is very knowledgeable about theater, politics, movies, and entertainers and feels successful when he can engage in discussions about information from prior to his stroke, as far back as his childhood.*

The mission of these groups is integration, wholeness, embracing the "new normal," acceptance of life changes, and a sense of spiritual healing, as well as improving communication, cognitive, and psychosocial skills and adapting to changes resulting from aphasia. This is achieved by helping the person with aphasia get the words out, make sense of jumbled language, and accept changes in life's path, in addition to connecting to a changed self and embracing in a different way all that was and still is.

It is this healing journey that has inspired me to create my program. I believe in the continuance of hope, energy, and holistic care. Too often the medical system fragments services and disregards the "whole person." The many voices reaching out for connection are my guide to respect and to help in the most humane way.

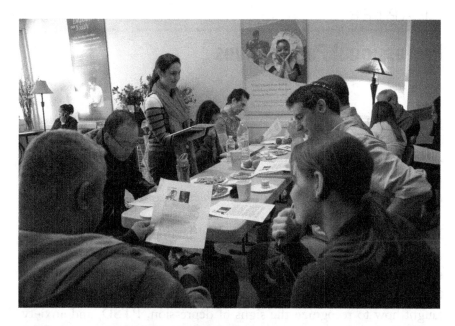

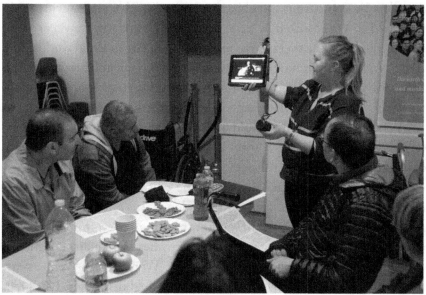

Individuals participating in groups

CHAPTER 3

Professional Perspectives

Social Work

For Mari Timpanaro, a social work intern in the Fall of 2013, her final internship at Metropolitan Communication Associates (MCA) proved to be the most professionally challenging and humbling experience.

If the eyes are the windows to the soul, then our observations are the stories that build the soul's memories. As practicing professionals in social work, we are taught to observe, to formulate, to build on the concrete congruency of theories in order to assess our clients. We are taught how to recognize the signs of depression, PTSD, and anxiety disorders by comparing the objective and subjective assessments with the DSM-5. We absorb how basic and complex empathy move, or stall, and how to build the therapeutic relationship between social worker and client. We are taught how best to understand our clients through verbal and non-verbal cues, but we are not taught how to guess. We are not taught how to interpret language when language goes missing.

When I learned that I would be working with persons with aphasia (PWAs) this year, it was a term that was unknown to me. I'd heard of apraxia, autism, and antisocial behaviors, but aphasia? Help! What were the signs of aphasia? What were the causes? How were we going to form a working relationship if the dialogue was one-sided? Would I go from being an intern who never quit speaking to becoming an intern who was mute? Was I going to be in over my head? So many questions, so few immediate answers. Even with the "World Wide Web" at my fingertips and e-mail conversations with my field instructor, I still felt ill-prepared. I'd learned that aphasia is a communication disorder that occurs after a person suffers a stroke or brain trauma and impairs a person's ability to process language, to speak, and to understand others.

I learned that aphasia is not a loss of intelligence; it just happens to be a diagnosis that impairs the ability to speak, read and/or write. The real work, the gratifying work, occurs after a person suffers their stroke and allows us into their lives. The work is learning about our clients from their perspective—how they see themselves in their family and community interactions. How would it be possible to learn a patient's past experiences to help address their current functioning if each of us had no idea what the other was saying?

I guess you could say these amazing people put me in my place quickly. All of these worries vanished over my first weeks. I learned that I had been assuming too much, that I was guilty of identifying them through their disability, not through their strength of character. Although they are different now from the people they used to be, they have an unwavering desire to be the best new self they can be. They insist on retaining as much of their former selves as possible and work tirelessly to regain new words and to better articulate their speech. They willingly open up their pasts to social workers like me by finding and connecting with the parts of our lives that bind us all together. These patients are daily reminders of what true inspiration and heroism means. Their stroke or traumatic brain injury altered their lives so completely, yet they persevere with humor and gratitude. We are just their sounding board, their idea catcher. They make the magic.

For Melissa DeLong, a social work intern in the Fall of 2013, working with her patients with aphasia opened her mind and continued to open her caring heart to the endless possibilities of human connection.

During my time as a therapist at Metropolitan Communication Associates (MCA), the clients often mentioned the indiscriminate nature of aphasia: it can happen to anyone. Aphasia arrives undeservedly and, typically, unexpectedly. Though at first this may seem sad, a deeper understanding brings to light the potential optimism of living with aphasia. This quality of aphasia is at once humbling and unifying—humbling in its blunt unveiling of the fragility of our mortal experience as humans, unifying in its ubiquity, its fairness, and its ability to bring together those affected. The potential for aphasia to impact any life is not something that is necessarily fretted about among the clients at MCA. Rather, it is simply stated. All life is allied in its temporality. Aphasia is yet another reminder of this. The women and men affected have become acquainted with life's unpredictability and temporality earlier than some, for sure, but this very fact has, though not without difficulty, fueled their lives. As a byproduct, it has fueled mine too.

After working at MCA, I came to understand that aphasia is not something the clients resent (at least not all of the time). On the contrary, many of them experience gratitude, not in spite of, but because of their aphasia, explaining how it has rendered them wiser, stronger, and more humane than was possible before. One client mentioned a higher level of consciousness and a sense of interconnectedness with others and with the world at large that was achieved as a result of aphasia's impediment on his ability to work. He described this deep level of connection being unattainable before, while in the midst of the distractions of everyday life and feeling the superficial pressures of society. I cannot speak to their lives prior to living with aphasia, but I can, with confidence, convey my belief in the unique strength, empathy, and awareness they have demonstrated post-aphasia. They bring with them the grit and determination that catalyzed and sustained their varied careers and relationships pre-aphasia, combined with a sensitivity for and compassion toward all others. From what I have witnessed, it is largely this combination that bolsters the understanding present during group therapies at MCA. The clients do not deny the inherent challenges that accompany aphasia, but encourage one another in the process of facing and overcoming those that are surmountable. And those that are not? Well, they know, perhaps better than many, that to accept one's limitations is not to be weak. It is not to give up. It is to celebrate our humanness, to laugh at it, to have compassion for it, and to find, whenever possible, ways to work around it. The clients at MCA are remarkable in their ability to do all of these things and have left a permanent and wonderful mark on my heart.

For Kim Singh, a social work intern in the Fall of 2013, her journey with aphasia began unexpectedly with family. Through her professional education, her journey has grown.

I had no idea what aphasia was prior to my brother's stroke. As a matter of fact, I refused to think that at 43 years old, my brother Mike, who is an exercise addict and the most health-conscious person in the family, was having a stroke. After almost four years, the struggles are still here, but it has definitely gotten much better in terms of dealing with the everyday challenges.

I have tried to embrace life no matter what it throws at me. When Mike survived his stroke, I considered it a miracle but never gave much thought to the person that I would become. Everyone knows how an unexpected sickness can change one's life forever. It was a beautiful Labor Day weekend when I received the call from my brother's wife that they were on their way to the hospital. Mike was having a very bad headache and had shown signs of slurred speech. That was it! From there everything just went downhill, at least until we heard that the surgery to prevent further brain damage was successful. The next few weeks were filled with round the clock hospital visits, arrangements, and consultations with doctors. Mike's severe brain damage had left him with the inability to speak, read, write, or walk.

After four weeks of rehabilitation, Mike left the hospital with the use of a walker and impaired communication due to aphasia. Home became an even more hectic place, juggling taking turns caring for my brother with the commitment of being a student. Many nights I looked up at the ceiling with my eyes filled with tears, unable to fall asleep, because I longed for the brother that I used to know. It took me a while before I finally understood that I had not lost my brother, but had simply been too overwhelmed with the changes. The most challenging of all was the fact that we couldn't communicate like before. There were times when I could not understand what he was trying to say, no matter how hard he tried. It was a difficult journey, but overtime my frustrations gave way to patience, understanding, and empathic communication.

Taking care of someone with aphasia is no easy thing to do, especially when you hardly know anything about the disorder. After I learned that I would be working with individuals with aphasia as part of my internship, I knew that I would fit right in. My caregiving experience and the little I knew about aphasia was helpful as I began working on a professional level. When I looked around at the individuals that I worked with, it certainly made it easier to understand that anybody can be affected with aphasia, and that lives can be changed forever. It's funny, but sometimes I wish I could turn back the hands of time to life without aphasia, when my brother was strong and active and would talk non-stop. Today, I am grateful for all the opportunities that I have been given to learn about the disorder. I am in a much better place because I was fortunate to be placed in an internship that really allowed me to see the bigger picture of aphasia and its impacts. My brother's strong will and determination to walk, read, write, drive, and speak again have given me hope, because day after day I witness his continued improvement.

For Amy Samelson, LMSW, her career in interior design ultimately lead her into a career as a clinical social worker. "I was missing the helping aspect of my work; I worked with people, but it wasn't complete for me," she says.

I did not truly come to understand aphasia until I met Mona Greenfield PhD, LCSW, CCC-SLP. As she intended it, the intimate therapeutic relationships I formed with the people whose lives were inextricably altered by stroke would teach me to understand the many faces of aphasia.

The best place to begin is with how a therapist can communicate with a client whose problem is speech impairment. Creativity is in play, and this is where it gets interesting. Two people with good will and intention, wishing to reach one another, work to find ways to reach out. Sometimes single words, drawings, pictograms, written words (when possible), guesswork on the part of the therapist (when permitted by the client), and pantomime are part of the new language. In process, stories are built, emotions are expressed and exchanged, and therapeutic bonds are formed.

Emotions are deeply affected by aphasia. As much as we all have them, for those who have had a stroke these emotions are unlike what you and I understand to be normal reactions. Frustration, temper, anger, tears, and depression, these are all mental states that come more easily with aphasia. I can only describe them as being somewhat closer to the surface, more available and more intense. In addition, clients with previous mental incapacities exhibit a kind of cross weave of symptoms made up of "what is and what was." This complicates the mental health picture.

It has been critical for me to develop slowness, patience, listening skills, and an increasing, sustainable empathy. It is equally important to understand that one should only replace words for those who struggle with them when asked. In this way, they retain their individual, self-determined right to communicate—a right we all have, whether we have been faced with disability or not.

Speech-Language Pathology

From a speech pathology intern to a primary therapist, Nicole Apostolou, MS, CCC-SLP, shares her impressions and experiences about aphasia.

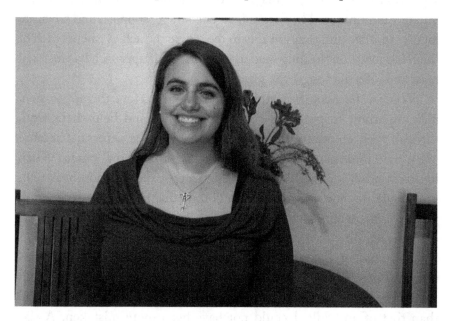

What is aphasia? Incredibly, most people have never hear of it unless it directly impacts a family member or close friend. For me, it is more than a loss of ability to understand or express speech; it is a role that you find yourself suddenly thrust into, and, as the lead actor, you are missing 90% of the script. It is a frightening experience, not only for the person suffering from aphasia, but also for the caregivers and family as well. Treatment and rehabilitation for aphasia can be a confusing process.

In schools and pediatric settings, a team approach is often encouraged. When a plan is put together, a teacher, social worker, physical therapist, occupational therapist, speech-language pathologist, psychologist and caregiver all collaborate to create goals and a therapeutic plan of care that is best for the child. Unfortunately, for adults that model is often lost upon discharge from the hospital or rehabilitation center, leaving patients and their caregivers without a cohesive plan. Through Metropolitan Communication Associates (MCA), we are fortunate to offer a setting where patients, care givers, aides, speech-language pathologists and social workers are able to create an individualized plan of care. In addition to their individual therapies, patients are able to attend cognitive groups, as well as relaxation and support groups. Through this practice, patients have formed their own micro communities. They are able to encourage, support, and advocate for one another, and they are able to recognize the achievements each of them has made on the long road to recovery. This approach has fostered trust and safety amongst the group.

When a client comes in stressed and emotional for a therapy session, it is important to put your counseling hat on and help them work through their emotions and problem solve. This is necessary because when the mind is stressed it enters into "fight or flight" mode. When in this mindset it is difficult to attend to a task and retain information, thus rendering one's therapeutic session ineffective. In my experience, when this team approach is used, we see the best outcomes by creating an understanding environment.

As a student, the adult population was not something I gravitated toward. Pediatrics appeared to present more challenges, and I thought I would be able to make a more significant impact in the life of a child than that of an adult. I could not have been more mistaken. A six-month internship led me down a completely different path—a path I am glad that I chose. Each therapy session presents its own struggles and challenges. As a therapist I am always happy to see and point out the gains each client has made. This can often be bittersweet, because although a client is happy to make progress toward more meaningful and functional communication, it is still not as perfect as he/she used to be. This is where a supportive and understanding attitude is needed to remind clients that their emotional response is warranted, but the acknowledgement of their successes is still relevant. I always emphasize to our clinical staff that we are treating the whole individual, not just their voice. With that mindset in place, our overarching goal is to improve our clients' overall quality of life by helping them achieve a functional normalcy and giving them the confidence they need to succeed in their day-to-day living.

For speech pathology intern Karen Han, the textbook details of aphasia could not compare to the in-person experiences she had while working with her patients.

Working in both individual and group therapy settings at Metropolitan Communication Associates (MCA) with individuals who have aphasia has been a wonderful and uniquely beneficial experience. It is truly inspirational to witness the resiliency, motivation, and hard work the clients consistently exhibit; they are engaged, focused, and always willing to volunteer and participate in the various planned activities and exercises. As a graduate student, I entered into my internship with certain expectations based on textbook scenario knowledge of the signs and symptoms of aphasia; however, the complexity of aphasia surprised me as I began to see firsthand that it is not a disorder that can be categorized into a simple grid, as no two clients exhibit the same symptoms. Each client displays different strengths and abilities that can be channeled to conduct an efficient therapy session.

The positive and enthusiastic participatory attitude of the clients, as well as the multidimensional aphasia programs facilitated by Dr. Greenfield, are what made my experience particularly noteworthy. At present, I am participating in the current events, literature, story, classical music, and trivia group therapy sessions. These sessions are the most rewarding and dynamic to experience, in the sense that I get a chance to watch the clients take part in discussions and, at times, have the privilege of observing a carry-over of skills they have been working on during individual therapy sessions. For example, during the story group therapy session, we discuss artwork by Pablo Picasso, Claude Monet, Paul Signac, and Leonardo Da Vinci. During this time, clients identify and relate to the beauty of the paintings by exploring ways to share how each particular piece of artwork makes them feel as they provide their personal interpretation of the painting. This time gives the clients an opportunity and a platform to explore, reflect, and express their thoughts.

I find the literature group—during which the clients will read a play together, analyzing and discussing the storyline and development of characters—to be one of the most vibrant group therapy sessions. During this time, not only are the clients working on intonation and prosody while reading the play, but they are also expressing their interpretation of the characters through acting. While reading and discussing the literature, clients share their feelings and understanding of how the play relates to their lives and how they find humor in the dialogue.

One of the most significant lessons I have learned while interning at MCA is that while I am working with clients who have aphasia, aphasia does not define who they are, nor should it limit the way they express themselves. I have come to appreciate the value and effectiveness of tapping into the clients' strengths through various modalities to provide them with individualized outlets for communication.

Nursing

Susan Bluhm, RN, shares her perspectives on aphasia as a nursing professor and from a personal perspective.

As a new nurse, I knew about speech problems that sometimes followed a stroke, but I hadn't experienced working with patients who had speech impairments yet. It was only when I became a nursing staff educator at a skilled nursing facility that I learned the term-aphasia. I remember she had thick, black, beautiful hair, and when the Certified Nursing Assistant (CNA) came over to brush her hair, she lit up. I realized that she could not talk; she could not make her wishes be known. I thought that was absolutely horrible, not being able to talk. A nurse co-worker said she had aphasia.

I eventually became a nursing professor at the local Community College and the Director of the CNA program. CNAs and many others in the medical field—including doctors, nurses, and allied health professionals—care for patients who have aphasia. Sometimes the students have little to no knowledge about aphasia. In the classroom, I go over the textbook definition, which is a "total or partial loss of the ability to use or understand language" caused when the parts of the brain responsible for language are damaged. I emphasize that any number of things can cause brain damage, including strokes, trauma, infection, cancer, and that there are different types of aphasia.

The textbooks only tell us the facts, which are a start, but they are purely clinical—very black and white without touching on the heart of the matter. Many people with aphasia are frightened, frustrated, alone, angry, and experiencing a host of other emotions. I ask my students, "What would it feel like to tell somebody something, but they couldn't understand a word you are saying? What would it feel like to try to get something across, but it wouldn't come out of our mouths? Or if it did come out, it wasn't what we wanted to say? Sometimes it could be backward, i.e. room bath, instead of bathroom."

What is missing from the textbook readings is the human heart. I show the students different ways they can facilitate communication, including letter boards, pictures, etc. After that, I emphasize the human element, having empathy and kindness, and I encourage students to take the time to talk to patients who have aphasia. I encourage students to *see* the longing to express their desires. Many patients with aphasia make a huge effort to talk, to convey meaning, and anyone who is really looking with compassion, can see the effort and let them know they see the struggle.

Even after the students know the textbook definition of aphasia, I find that some CNA students ignore patients, at least until they get to know them. In my experience, many students feel very sorry for these patients. They are very judgmental of the "experienced" nurses and other CNAs regarding their apparent indifference to the patients. The students feel the CNAs are not as attentive, helpful, or understanding as they should be. Of course when those "experienced" CNAs were students they said the same thing.

At this point a discussion ensues regarding patience—about how difficult is it not only for the patient with aphasia, but also for the caregiver. What can a caregiver do? What attributes might a caregiver have? What is the difference between empathy and sympathy?

A particular student saw a patient sitting for hours, not able to talk. He went over to the patient and just sat with him, then looked him in the eyes and asked him how he was really doing. The patient picked up his head, stared right back at the student and smiled. They were able to communicate, albeit with difficulty. The student was extremely patient, focused, and caring, and the patient responded.

If students take the time to see the human element, the struggles and eventual advances and successes (sometimes in very small increments), they will be able to see a full human being, with the same hopes, desires, and individual personalities as before the aphasia.

I encourage the students to talk to other healthcare team members (speech therapists, occupational therapists, etc.) for ideas on how to communicate, and to enlist family members and friends who know them well. There are many clever ideas that CNAs use to communicate: picture boards, letter boards, and yes and no signs. In addition to communication strategies, I tell students that there are other important things to think about:

- The patient is not doing this deliberately to bother you.
- The patient may be angry at the situation, and you are the closest person she or he has to take it out on.
- Life is not always fair.
- Everything the patient knew and took for granted is gone.
- Empower the patient as much as possible (e.g. give choices).

When I was a new nurse, my own experience with aphasia became highly personal. In her late 60s, my mother began to have muscle weakness. It turned out it was ALS. I had barely heard the word "aphasia" and certainly thought it was something that happened to "others," never anybody I knew. Although ALS does not fit the textbook definition of aphasia, my mother's muscles that were used for speech weakened and deteriorated until she lost the ability to speak at all. (ALS often does not affect the ability to type or read, until advanced).

I learned that life has a way of humbling us very quickly, life has a way of connecting us to one another, and life has a way of helping us find the common denominator in each of us. As Oscar Wilde said, "Anything human is not alien to me."

Many years later, my daughter had a stroke and resulting aphasia at age 41. By that time, I knew all about the loss of communication through speech. At first, she could not speak at all. After a couple of months, she started to speak but was hard to understand. I sat in on one speech therapy session, and it was a good thing I did. She is a perfectionist and very hard on herself, constantly repeating words for better, clearer articulation. Her speech therapist emphasized that it is all about conveying meaning in conversation, and if listeners understand what you say the first time, you do not have to repeat the words. I felt that it interrupted the flow of conversation and was glad to find support from the speech therapist.

CHAPTER 4

Aphasia and the Arts

Ellayne S. Ganzfried, MS, CCC-SLP

Mona Greenfield, PhD, LCSW, CCC-SLP

Aphasia therapy through the arts provides an enriching milieu to facilitate communication skills. Listening, speaking, reading, and writing can all be enhanced through art. There is substantial literature attesting to the benefits of music and art therapies for persons with aphasia (PWAs) (Hobson, 2006; Peterson, 2006).

Aphasia groups and centers share the goal to help individuals live successfully with aphasia. Benefits of groups include meeting others with aphasia, establishing friendships, building self-confidence, and accessing a supportive, communicative environment that offers meaningful educational and recreational activities (Elman, 2007). Listening, speaking, reading, and writing are all important aspects of aphasia treatment. Through the arts, all of these skills can be integrated into therapy providing a motivating and humanizing experience for patients with aphasia. The skills addressed in individual therapy sessions are generalized, or applied, through a range of activities involving group art presentations and discussion groups. Traditionally, drawing has been incorporated into therapy as a communication aid to help patients with severe aphasia improve communication, improve participation, and retain social membership (Rao, 1995; Ward-Lonergan & Nicholas, 1995). Utilization of the unimpaired right brain has also been effective for some patients in stimulating language in Melodic Intonation Therapy (Sparks & Holland, 1976).

A unique collaboration has been established between the National Aphasia Association (NAA) and the Museum of Modern Art (MoMA) in NYC, in which the museum offers the opportunity for local aphasia groups to visit and receive guided tours. The strength of this program is built upon the relationship between the docent and the aphasia group, which is created through a three-pronged approach. The docent attends the aphasia group prior to the scheduled visit to provide an overview of the artist and exhibition that will be viewed. This prompts group discussion and the expression of individual thoughts and opinions related to the pieces they will be viewing. The group then visits the museum exhibition to view the work that was previously discussed. Lastly, the docent attends the group afterwards as a follow-up to gain impressions and insights that group members express after viewing the collection. The docent uses the work that was exhibited as a springboard to facilitate discussion of the artwork and to have the group members create their own art. There is also potential for the work created by the PWAs to be featured in community art exhibitions organized by the museum. The work done at the MoMA is carried over into weekly therapy through an art group in which an artist or therapy prompt linked to emotions or a topic is given, and the group is given time to create their own vision linked to the prompt. Afterwards group members are given an opportunity to share information about their pieces. The results of this program have been notable, with documented increased communication attempts, interactions, and discovery of artistic talents.

Through the arts, these PWAs are given an opportunity to draw and paint within a communicative milieu fostered by this normalizing experience. For PWAs, skills including word finding, describing information, people and events, processing information, recalling information, producing speech, organizing new knowledge learning, drawing inferences, and problem solving are stimulated through creative processes in a gratifying and naturalistic communicative context.

Utilizing the arts with persons with aphasia empowers participants by allowing everyone to take part, regardless of aphasia severity, physical impairment, or previous experience. It affords an opportunity for a group of PWAs to collaborate, coach, and support each other during activities.

Family, friends, and caregivers benefit by seeing their loved one's range of capabilities. Participation encourages spontaneous communication in a relaxed and predictable environment. Opportunities to communicate using various modalities and communication strategies are provided. Participation provides the PWA the opportunity to discover a new talent, learn a new skill, or return to a valued, meaningful activity.

This translates to gains in linguistic, psycho-social, emotional, and recreational skills.

A classroom collaboration at the MoMA was also established through this program. PWAs attended five sessions with the art educator to tour the museum and create art in the museum classroom. Caregivers, aides, and clinicians all participated. Each week a different type of art was created by all, including collage, ink paintings, sculpture with clay, water color, and drawing.

During the session, the educator gave the participants a prompt, and then they created works that reflected their sense of themselves. Many of these works were indirectly about aphasia. One participant commented about a large head in his painting, saying, "This is aphasia." The opportunity to do this work at the MoMA was powerful and normalizing. Many exhibits by groups who did work in the classroom were displayed and our group was very proud to be considered for this option in the future.

After work was completed each week, there was a discussion about each participant's work. The sharing and comments about each other's work not only facilitated communication but was also an amazing social experience and chance to feel well-integrated in the community.

The participants were not only characterized by "aphasia," they were artists, observers, and storytellers. They were part of sharing and enjoying the MoMA with the crowds of visitors and tourists sharing, enjoying, and living together. Through this experience, a sense of normalcy was created. Participants felt like others who visit the MoMA and discuss art. In the passages that follow, some of the participants share their reactions to being part of this amazing collaboration.

Gordon Sasaki, MoMA Educator

As an independent contract MoMA educator, I have had the opportunity to work with Mona's group in collaboration with the National Aphasia Association (NAA) for approximately seven years now and have witnessed remarkable growth in many of her long time participants.

I have been working in the area of arts access for almost twenty-five years now as an artist/educator. My academic and studio training are supported by a personal relationship with disability after a 1982 automobile accident, which injured my spine and resulted in the need of a wheelchair for basic mobility. Like most, my initial medical care was to diagnose and treat acute physical injury almost as a separate entity from the psycho-emotional wellbeing of the patient. My natural curiosity as an artist and an interest for a clearer understanding of why my legs no longer worked, led me to a more in-depth study of physiology. But the more I studied the body, the more I became aware of the body as something more than a moving, breathing, organism. I began to understand it also as a container of meaning and extension of the self. It became clear to me that for true understanding and communication to take place, we need to approach any individual as a holistic being regardless of ability.

This is where my art training has become invaluable. Arts plasticity as a tool is remarkable in its ability to wrap itself around the needs of the individual; rather than forcing a one-way approach, it has many equally valid access points. This flexibility allows each user to take in, interpret, and express their personal experience in numerous modalities. Whether through movement, sound, speech, writing, drawing, sculpture, etc., art has an inherent ability to stimulate human expression and to adapt itself towards interaction and communication. This is where we began.

For this particular aphasia group, some of our common fundamental goals were to use the arts as a vehicle to make connections and promote therapeutic conversation, thus helping to redevelop the language and speech skills of the participants and enriching their overall lives through social interaction and community engagement.

With a general understanding that disability, in this case aphasia, has the potential of impacting anyone, regardless of age, race, gender, or social or economic status, as expected, the diversity of Mona's group reflects this fact. While all in this group are adults, participants range greatly in age, profession, art and life experience, and even degrees of impairment. This diversity emphasizes the need to address the individual needs and interests of each person in order to make engaging and meaningful connections. After all, art may not be the center of everyone's lives, but creativity has benefits that apply to all aspects of life.

Our approach has been to generally arrange two partnerships a year, with consideration to appropriateness and interest in particular exhibitions. Each partnership is composed of three 90-minute sessions. In session one, I visit the group to introduce the artworks through reproductions and discussion. In session two, we visit the museum to actually view and experience the works first hand, keeping in mind that like any public venue any museum can sometimes be a loud and boisterous place with many challenges, especially from the perspective of an individual with impaired communication skills. In the last session, we meet to discuss individual interpretations and experiences of the session at the museum. This provides the opportunity to deepen the discussion and understanding of the artwork or previous visit, and includes any tangential connections that individuals discover between art and their daily lives.

In 2014, we began an extended partnership, where the approach was to meet for a total of five 2-hour sessions and to use the time more as a hands-on artist studio, actually making artwork.

During this extended partnership, we began with the theme of the "self-portrait," using familiar and basic materials like pencil and paper. We took nothing for granted and did not assume that individuals had any previous experience. From this starting point we developed more complex approaches through a variety of mediums, scaffolding (or building techniques from previous sessions), and ending in sculptural busts. Each session concluded with a viewing of the created artwork with discussion and reflection by the artists.

While not focusing on the end goal of creating "masterworks" of art during these sessions, many of the works are, in fact, remarkable in their aesthetic sincerity, certainly felt by even the untrained eye. These personal art expressions become excellent subjects to encourage discussion and engage the participants at another level of connection and dialog. By emphasizing this process of creative discovery, participants are encouraged to expand their abilities into artistic territories that they previously may have found intimidating and to express themselves through a potentially new visually-based language. Through the process of discussion, participants develop new art vocabulary and practice verbalizing abstract ideas and thoughts about their works.

Ultimately, all of these approaches are intended to reflect our common overall goals of helping to find a sense of normalcy and well-being for each person, with the understanding that normalcy doesn't have to mean life as it used to be or a pursuit of something unattainable that society defines as normal. Most important is a respectful approach that acknowledges the individual needs and challenges of the disability, aphasia or otherwise, and directs energy into healing the entire person, both body and soul.

While art can at times be challenging on many levels, at others raw and heart-wrenchingly sincere, one aspect of art that often fails to get mentioned is that art can also be a lot of fun. Fun as a practical tool for engagement can sometimes be underestimated in the clinical environment. Often accompanied with fun is humor and laughter, and all are important components of each of our daily make-up and who we are as human beings. All of these can easily be incorporated into the discussion of artists and the making of artworks.

Fran

We went to the MoMA with Gordon. Gordon gave a tour of the museum. I enjoyed the tour because it was special, and it made me feel normal to do something like that. In the classroom he taught us about art, and we did an art project with clay. I made a self-portrait out of the clay. We also made collages. I remember Gordon's sculpture had a lot of hair. I felt alive being in the classroom making art again. Learning in the museum made me feel like I was in school again because I studied art in college.

Aaron

(Written with the assistance of his speech pathologist, Nicole Apostolou, MS, CCC-SLP.)

I have always had a passion for art, and I appreciate it in all its forms. Visiting the MoMA is one of my favorite things to do. Having the opportunity to go to the MoMA to be a part of the program there was great. I was able to create different types of art with my friends from group and with Tracy, my wife. One of my paintings in particular is important to me. It shows the day I had my stroke in an abstract way. I call the painting, "One Day." It is the moment where the neurons in my brain disconnected. Now, I am working on building those connections once again. In another drawing, I tried to capture the famous conductor Gustavo Dudamel and his orchestra. I feel that listening to music and making or looking at art are a great release. Since my stroke, language and speech can be difficult. I sometimes feel overwhelmed and frustrated because of this. But, music and art don't require words and it helps me relax. My experience at the MoMA was a validating experience, and it allowed me to further explore my love of art and make connections with those around me.

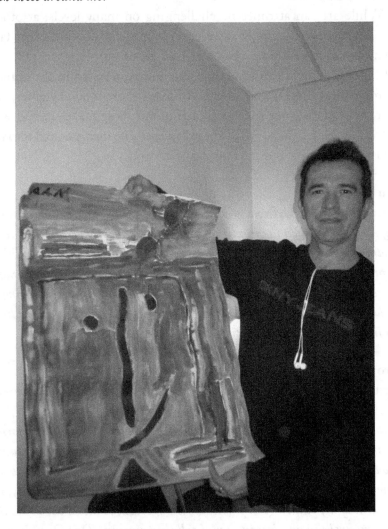

CHAPTER 5

The Power of Storytelling

Ellayne S. Ganzfried, MS, CCC-SLP

Mona Greenfield, PhD, LCSW, CCC-SLP

"For we dream in narrative, daydream in narrative, remember, anticipate, hope, despair, believe, doubt, plan, revise, criticize, construct, gossip, learn, hate, and love by narrative. In order really to live, we make up stories about ourselves and others, about the personal as well as the social past and future" (Hardy, 1978, p.13).

Literature from the social sciences situates narrative as a fundamental life concern of humans (Shadden & Hagstrom, 2007). Personal narratives have been used as a successful strategy for persons with aphasia (PWAs) serving many functions including (1) the reconstruction of one's identity and sense of self (Shadden & Hagstrom, 2007), (2) the establishment of social relationships (Davidson, Worrall, & Hixon, 2008), and (3) the formation of a hopeful future life (Bright, Kayes, McCann, & McPherson, 2013). Narrative provides the opportunity to engage in increasing participation in authentic communicative contexts that offer supports within the speaker's community and increases confidence and a positive sense of self (Simmons-Mackie, N., 2001). Yet, Hinckley (2008) explains that using narrative development as the focus of direct communication treatment is not a common practice by speech-language pathologists.

Producing a cohesive narrative can be challenging for PWAs due to the language processing and production issues consistent with aphasia. Narratives require the integration of cognitive skills, syntax, semantics, articulation, and pragmatic skills. PWAs are often reticent to produce narratives as they struggle to organize information and find the words to tell their stories. However, the opportunity to share these stories in a group can be a normalizing experience and facilitate participation in the larger social community. The majority of work in aphasic discourse tends to look at discourse involving picture descriptions, story retell, and procedural discourse. These all involve language focused on the third-person that is removed from the life experiences of PWAs, topics familiar or interesting to them, or their (possibly emotionally tinged) attitudes (Fromm et al., 2011). Social models in aphasia assessment and treatment, though less frequently used, do encourage the inclusion of personally relevant experience in the assessment and treatment of aphasia. While there has been investigation of the benefits of telling personal stroke narratives in aphasia therapy, there has not been extensive exploration of the impact of self-determined narratives that are not directly related to the impairment.

To this end, the collaboration initiated between The Moth and a local aphasia program—Metropolitan Communication Associates (MCA)—provided a unique opportunity for PWA to create, practice, and develop competence in storytelling outside of the typical clinician/client intervention model. The Moth (www.themoth.org) is an acclaimed not-for-profit organization. The Moth's mission is to promote the art and craft of storytelling and to honor and celebrate the diversity and commonality of human experience. Since its launch in 1997, The Moth has presented thousands of stories told live and without notes. Through ongoing programs in more than 25 cities, The Moth has presented over 18,000 stories to standing-room-only crowds worldwide and it currently produces more than 500 live shows each year. Moth shows are renowned for the great range of human experience they showcase. Since each story is true and every voice authentic, the shows dance between documentary and theater, creating a unique, intimate, and often enlightening experience for the audience. Moth stories dissolve socio-economic barriers, expose vulnerabilities, and quietly suggest ways to overcome challenges and see with new eyes. This philosophy correlates with the evidence that resilience matters for PWA (Hinckley, 2006; Holland, 2010), and that therapy that includes a focus on resilient behaviors can especially help in aphasia where communication skills are involved (Fromm et al., 2011).

The Moth Community Program offers workshops and performance opportunities to people who are under-represented in mainstream media or feel under-heard. The program teaches participants how to shape selected life experiences into well-crafted stories and share them with members of their communities and beyond. Eight PWAs participated in a pilot Moth Community Workshop. They were coached by Moth program facilitators, with speech-language pathology students serving as communication supports for the PWAs. Several sessions initially focused on developing rapport and trust. Participants were provided with examples of stories and guided through exercises using a workbook in story construction. These exercises provided the framework for creating, organizing, scripting, and rehearsing their stories. The workshop culminated in a storytelling event for friends and families that was videotaped and shared.

It was a very interesting collaboration; no one knew exactly what to expect. How would the participants do at communicating their stories when language and speaking are exactly the challenges with aphasia? It turned out that most storytellers experienced moments of being caught up and engaged with the stories themselves, instead of focusing on the difficulties encountered trying to express the stories. The Moth project empowered these PWAs to share a piece of themselves in a group environment free of judgment. It allowed them to focus less on the "perfection of production" and more on attitudes, emotions, and nonverbal/paralinguistic skills like gesture, body language, facial expressions, intonation, rate, and stress patterns. The response to this program was overwhelmingly positive. Participants reported improved confidence, self-esteem, self-awareness, and a renewed identification with "normalcy." It was a refocusing on who they are and their experiences with a sense of humor and vulnerability. They appeared more willing to communicate spontaneously and create deeper connections within their community. We asked the Moth coaches to share their experiences.

Larry Rosen, Moth Community Program Manager

Did you have previous knowledge of aphasia?
I did not have previous knowledge. I knew there were communication difficulties that often followed strokes but was unfamiliar with aphasia as a defined condition.

What were your expectations in working with individuals with aphasia?
I honestly had no expectations. I felt we were well-prepared,

knowledge-wise, based on our initial meeting with Ellayne. But I had no idea how we how we would feel meeting and working with participants.

What were the greatest challenges?

Seriously, the greatest challenges were not aphasia-related. Instead they were the challenges we often face with people in any workshop: a reticence or resistance to revealing oneself emotionally, the discipline called-for in crafting, telling, and retelling the story, etc.

What did and didn't work in facilitating stories?

It was all about patience. The more we slowed down our work pace, and the more we tamed our excitement (and urgency), in regards to "getting the story," the happier we all were.

What did you learn from working with this group?

Again, what differed most from other Community Workshops was the pace at which we worked. Once we extended the time frame beyond our accustomed six weeks (actually doubling it), we were all better able to relax into and enjoy the process.

How did this experience differ from other community workshops?

I came away from this workshop more aware than ever that the things that unite us all as humans – our feelings, relationships, passions, and experiences – far outweigh and outnumber the things that make us different.

What makes storytelling so universally appealing?

I believe what makes Moth storytelling – i.e., the sharing of true, personal stories – so appealing is our fascination with (and, ideally, empathy for) the lives of others, combined with an innate fascination with narrative.

How did you feel individuals with aphasia engaged in the Moth process?

Once trust was established (it took a few sessions), they engaged well, and we all had a great time working together. In this way, again, it was like any other workshop.

Carly McCollow, Moth Community Workshop Coach

Before working with the National Aphasia Association (NAA), I did not know what aphasia was, even though there was someone in my family struggling with it. No one in my family had heard of that term. Once we understood what was happening with our family member, and I began working with the NAA through The Moth, we were able to begin approaching the situation differently, with more understanding and compassion.

My expectations working with those with aphasia were that they would have difficulty recalling and speaking words. What I was not expecting were the myriad of ways that aphasia can uniquely challenge each individual. Once I understood the techniques that each individual had created to unlock their speech and language recall, I was much better able to facilitate the communication process. Each individual and I created different techniques and signals for how I could help them through a difficult moment: waiting, handing them pen and paper, trying to fill in the blank, guessing the words they could mean that started with a letter, reading the letters they shaped with their hands, words of encouragement, etc.

This workshop was different from other Moth workshops because of the way that the individuals had to overcome a compounded challenge— not just the self-reflection and self-expression required to conceive and craft a five minute story, but also the added challenge of doing so when language recall and speaking the language was a struggle. Some of these individuals also found it more difficult to speak when they were experiencing stress or anxiety, and while the environment in the room during the workshop was supportive and easy, they encountered this anxiety about publicly sharing their stories with the full group. It was an incredible experience to watch them stand up and take the floor to speak their stories. It was an incredible display of courage and resilience.

Janet Kim, Moth Community Workshop Coach

Before this workshop, I had never even heard of aphasia, and when I first heard about this opportunity, I felt in truth daunted by the challenge but extremely moved by the possibilities. Even working with people with full command of their communications abilities, the process of crafting a story can be very difficult for a number of reasons: from the first step of keying in on truly meaningful moments and memories and experiences and being able to distill their significance, to then trying to find the right words to convey that powerfully to an audience, and then to be able to recall it and repeat it.

As an instructor, I also was concerned about whether I'd be able to understand everyone; how would we communicate together to build these stories? Would I be putting words into people's mouths (the greatest no-no for any group we work with)? How could I "listen" if communication itself could be challenging? If someone told a different story one session from the next, or different details, was it because the previous one was not important, or was it due to memory recall challenges associated with aphasia?

One of the things that working with this group reinforced for me was how important and invaluable a strong community can be. Everyone was so supportive of one another (and were just awesome individuals), which I think greatly facilitated the process. I think that one-on-one time was helpful, as well as working in even smaller groups, with more time. Repetition was key, and I think that notes and visuals like the story map were especially useful and critical. Learning how to listen in different ways—like looking to see if Lindy perked up at a suggestion, or shook her head vigorously—and being patient and gentle about things without feeling bad about potential misunderstandings was important too. I think once we were able to identify the theme, or emotional heart of what each person wanted to express, it all flowed from there. And that's true of every group we work with.

I think it was wonderful, humbling, etc. to see how committed everyone was to the process, even after we tagged on all of those extra sessions, and, well, everyone had amazing stories to boot.

The Moth Storyteller Stories

The following stories were told live, and are transcribed verbatim below by Nicole Apostolou. Any errors are consistent with the individual's communication impairment:

Lindy

(As told with the aid of her iPad and her art book.)

When I was six years old I lived in Japan with my parents. I enjoyed living in Japan and felt connected to Japanese culture. While living in Japan, I got a present from my parents on Easter of 1952. The present was an origami book that I still have and cherish. [*Shows her origami book to the audience.*] I visited Japanese temples with my family. While on a visit to a temple in Japan, I crawled into a small crawl space. Above me was a statue of Buddha. When seeing Buddha, I had a rush of emotions, and I decided to become a Buddhist. It was a profound experience for my discovered Buddha. I began to feel inspired and surrounded by Buddha. After becoming a Buddhist, I developed feelings of strength, freedom, courage, confidence, and passion. Buddha became a pillar of strength for me throughout my life. Buddha is what helped me to be strong after my stroke.

When I had my stroke, I felt Buddha's presence come over me like a huge rush. It was just like the rush I felt as a child. It was amazing... wow. Then I realized that I could not move my right hand, arm, or leg. My right side was paralyzed. But I did not get scared or upset. Because of my faith in Buddha, I felt calm. It was going to be *okay*. I could also still feel my left side and move my left arm, which meant I could still paint. It was difficult at first, but I worked hard and did exercises to get stronger. Buddha gave me the strength and passion to continue to paint. and my faith became even stronger.

Fran

I met him at NYU. I was in NYU, and I went in, and there was a man, and he was very cute, and I thought I'd like to meet him, and he was talking to me, and then he said, "I gotta go." Next Friday, I was at NYU, and I came in, and he said, "Do you know how to dance?" So I said, "Yes," and I said, "Can you go out? Saturday night there is a dance and I can meet you." And he did, and he was really a good dancer. So then he was telling me about the artists. He was an artist. So I said, "I would like to go and see your sketches," and he says, "Oh, I'll show you, I've got a lot of things to show you." He came with all this stuff and it was beautiful... beautiful. And he was an artist. I was unusual. I liked the man. He went to Florida with me to see my Aunts. He liked it. That was two weeks, and then he went home.

Oh and the boxing! He showed me how to box. Oh, and he moved out into Flushing, and he met his girlfriend there. I stayed in touch with him. He still came to see me, not very often. He had seizures, many, many, many seizures. I stood by him. I had a seizure also. So, I watched him. His daughter called when he passed away, and she said, "Bud passed away. Can you come in tomorrow for the funeral?" I couldn't do it. I couldn't do it. I couldn't do it. I have memories. Good memories. He's always in my heart.

Lee

Before my demise, I did Tango for one year, and I liked it because I wanted to. I liked the music, and I liked the dance a lot, and so I did the Milonga, which is a very close embrace with your body, your upper body on your husband or something. I liked it, but when I had a stroke I couldn't do it. But five years since, I wanted to go and see what it was like any way, so I went to Milonga, which is a dance party. And so I went there, and I went and just watched, which is called sentado, which is mainly for the girls who don't know how to dance. But I did, but I couldn't do it anymore. But I went and just did a lot of sentado, and then I went to my dance instructor and said, "Do you think I could dance again?" And he said he thought I would. So I danced a lot with him, with a partner so that I could do it. And then I went to the Milonga again, but I didn't know.

But a lot of people, girls who didn't know what I was going through and didn't know the dance any way, didn't know that I was doing it wrong. And I did get a girl who said I was doing it not very well, and I said, "Well I'm glad you saw that, because I didn't know." And she said that because you don't do it with this (showing his fingers), you do it with this (showing his palm), and I was fading the background, but it should be here (demonstrating positioning of the hand on the upper torso). So I liked what she said, but I went to the sentado, and I stood back a lot so I could see what was going on with the position, and I've been doing it. I know the molinete, the enganche, the sandwichito and the cruzada, but I can't. I know it here (pointing at head), but I'm not doing it all the time, but I hope I will do it. If you can Tango, then you can do a lot of stuff.

Yvonne Honigsberg

My mother could be described in three words—histrionic, hysterical and high volume. But she was secretive—about the most important things. She never told anybody that her husband was an alcoholic; she never told anyone that she spent her childhood inside a refugee camp escaping from the Nazi's; and never told *me* that I was adopted.

When I was 14 years old, my mother was talking on the phone, and I heard something alarming. I raced into my bedroom and leapt up on my rainbow-colored bed, my heart pounding. She came to my room and stood in the doorway and said, "Yvonne, you were adopted." Suddenly, the roar inside my head was deafening. *(Said telegraphically.)* Chills were running up and down my spine. It was like a bomb or a nuclear holocaust had gone off or been dropped into my world, and I thought, I didn't know what to do. I thought, "What? You're not my mother? You're not my mother? Well, who is my mother then?"

I felt unmoored and lost. So, I made up my mind to search for my biological mother when I was 18 years old, because I thought that for sure nobody would tell me anything about my birth mother until I was "of age." So during the next 4 years, I searched for my mother in every face I saw that looked like me. During... um, when I turned 18 and I started my search the next day, and I found out that all the records were closed. The adoption records were closed in New Jersey, meaning that I could *never* find out anything about my birth mother and she would *never* find out *any* information about me!

So I thought, there is only one thing a person would do in my situation... I would have to break into the adoption agency under cover of the night—with flashlight in hand and pray *(play)* private eye! So, the next day I came to my senses and thought, hmm, maybe I should just call them and see what they had to say. I did, and they said "Come in and see a social worker," and I did. And the social worker said, "Okay, you want to look for your mother, but I must warn you: adopted people think that *their* mothers must be rich and ef-famous or both, but I can assure you, this is seldom the case! They might be poor, or drug addicts, or worse yet, they might not want to meet you. I said, "Okay, well... I'm willing to take the risk!

The next thing she said was, so, your birth mother has just called us last week, and she said if her daughter should ever come looking for her, t(*o*) open the records up *(f)*ully. So I was... wowed. So you mean it's going to be that easy? Wow. So *(s)*et up da meeting. *(slurred.)*

So, on the day of the meeting I was very, very nervous and I, I *(b)*urst into the door of the social workers office, and I saw her, and I thought, "Wow, she doesn't look anything like me. Maybe there's been some mistake?" And she was thinking, "She doesn't look anything like me... she looks exactly like her father." But they confirmed that they got it right. And Susan, that was her name, and was amazing. She was the polar opposite of my Mom. She was educated. She could talk with ease about, uh, lots of interesting *(s)*ubjects, art and politics, and she was funny and light. She traveled and, and was open-minded.

At the same time my mother didn't even graduate from high school, through no fault of her own, but still. She'd talk about the weather, the clothes I was wearing, and gossip, and she was always worried about something and anxious. So um, Susan and I developed a relationship. We would call each other, write letters to each other, and once in a while see each other. It was fabulous. Until... I never told any of this to my mother, cause I thought for sure she would feel hurt, betrayed, and threatened. And we didn't have that kind of open relationship. This went on for a couple of years.

Until one day when I was home from college during the summer, my sister confronted me in the bathroom, and she said, "Yvonne, are you a lesbian *(accusatory tone)?*" I said, "No. Why ever would you say that *(incredulous tone)?*" And she said, "Because... I found a letter from a women named Susan that said 'I miss you, I love you, I can't wait to see you again.' That's why!" For a moment, I thought about copping to being a lesbian. But I said, "Nooo. Oh my God, Susan is not my lesbian lover! She's my biological mother. She was... I was adopted." And my sister was stunned because she had never heard that before. She ran into my mother's room to confirm that it was true.

A few minutes later, my mother came to my room looking pale as a ghost, stood in the doorway and said, "Is it true? Did you meet your biological mother?" I say, "Yes, it true." She acted angry and hurt, and we didn't talk about it ever fully again. And there was a lot tension mounting in our relationship. It was like the big, fat elephant in the room.

Um, but, um, from time to time, my mother started asking me about Susan, like where she lived, what she did for a living, was she married, to which I answered her as quickly as possible. I squirmed at her inquiries and wanted to get off the subject right away. It was supposed to be *my* secret. I wanted to keep them suppur (*slurred–separate*).

But... Until one day my mother said to me, "Yvonne, I want to meet Susan." And I thought, "Oh... My... God... My two worlds are about to collide." But, but, I set up a meeting (*slurred*) very reluctantly. But um, so, and Susan live in Boston, and we live in New Jersey, so I set up a meeting at a restaurant in New Haven, CT. So, on the infamous day (*nervous laughter*), we went into the restaurant, and I introduced them, and they shook hands. And my mother was the first one to speak. She said, "Susan, I have something to tell you." And I cringed because I thought for sure she would say something humiliating or embarrassing or inappropriate for me, as she often did. And she said, "Susan, I want thank you so much for bringing Yvonne into this world. She is light of my life." (*Said with raw emotion and pointed confidence*). "You've given me such a gift in Yvonne. (*Silence.*)"

And I was shocked. I was stunned at her naked gratitude. There was no drama or fanfare... It was just warm and gracious and real.

So, um, we chatted and after our lunch, on our way we back to the car, we decided to share an ice cream cone—mint chocolate chip. And she took one lick. And I took one lick. And we sat... in silence, but it was a different sort of silence. It was a peaceful, warm, loving silence.

CHAPTER 6

Voices of Aphasia

For Al, this was a moment of time that changed the course of his life in ways he could never have imagined. As he shares candidly, "You can't make this stuff up."

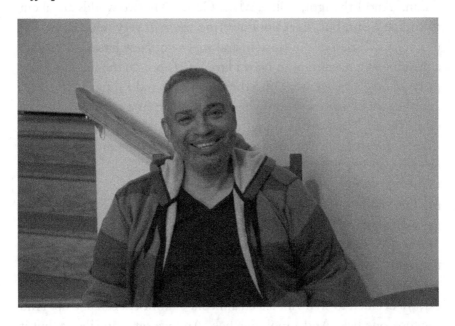

I woke up to go to work, and I felt strange. I tried to call my job, but I could not see the numbers. I ended up lying on the couch from 8:30 a.m. until late in the afternoon. I can't remember what time I tried to get up. Sometime after 9:00 a.m. I said to myself, "Well, I won't call my job now. It's too late." At that time, I was working for the Department of Buildings on Broadway and Chambers. I found my way into the bedroom and fell asleep. I heard the phone ringing at 4:20 p.m., but I couldn't move. It was my wife on the answering machine, saying that she was working overtime. I couldn't move to answer the phone. When

I first woke up that morning, I never had the presence of mind to call 911. It felt like an out of body experience all day. What I realize now, is that on that day *I was stroking*.

My wife came home at 8:30 p.m. and said, "What's up with you?" Noticing that I couldn't move and couldn't talk well, my wife called 911. The paramedics came and carried me down 36 steps in their chair. The ambulance stayed outside of my house for what felt like 10 minutes. I was on a stretcher on my way to the hospital.

My first night at the hospital, I hallucinated that a nurse stole a computer, and that they saw me watching them. I saw nurses praying to Buddha, and I thought they were trying to cut my hands and cut my testicles off. I still see nightmares of this male nurse to this day—him wearing red lipstick trying to warn me to keep quiet about all that I'd seen, or thought that I'd seen. I thought that the nurses were role playing, reading from a script, telling me I was faking my stroke. In my hallucination when the nurses changed shifts, there was a new nurse who was arguing with the other nurse, telling her to stop bothering me. The older nurse told the new nurse that they were just role playing and having fun. I really let my imagination run wild! It was out of control!

While at the hospital, it felt like a torture chamber. They inserted a breathing tube down each nostril. It was torture. And they suctioned me, a gross procedure where they scraped my tongue. *Yuck.* That was torture too. My wife was arguing with me in my hallucination, saying that I was a lazy son of a gun, who didn't want to help myself. One day, my whole family was visiting with me. I couldn't talk. I had a g-tube (gastro tube, like a feeding tube) and a breathing tube, and I felt like I was on a merry-go-round with this whole operation, this whole experience. To add to my already running imagination, I saw a nurse with a plastic arm. I saw ladies with parasols. I felt like a fool when the doctor told me, earnestly, that he wasn't fooled by me and my acting skills. I remember a male nurse and some of his buddies taking bets on when I would fall asleep. Just to mess with them, I'd fight my eyes getting heavy and open my eyes really wide to make him lose the bet. I remember a speech therapist saying that she couldn't work with me because I sounded like there was an exorcist-type monster inside me. I wished I was dead.

After my one month stay in the hospital, I was transferred over to the nursing home. I was there for six months. My first roommate would always tell my wife, my goddaughter, my sister and I how he killed people in Vietnam. I was crying hysterically the night he barricaded himself in the bathroom and the nurses had to come storming in to break down the door. What a scary night! After that night, they moved him to a private room on another floor, thank goodness. I was so thankful when they brought my new roommate to stay. He was quiet! He was German and spoke very little English, which helped me regain my sanity and composure. Too bad he didn't bring in borscht to share!

I remember every morning at the nursing home how the nurse would come in early and tell us to change our sleeping positions and wait until breakfast. She'd barge in, scream the order at us, then leave, making us fend for ourselves. What a nightmare. I knew I had to do something, for myself and for other patients. I called a representative from the insurance company, as well as a health inspector. Take that nursing home! I knew that something more had to be done to protect my sanity. I tried to escape. It was in the middle of winter, and with no winter coat, I made a break for the door. The guard questioned me, asking, "Where are you going?!"

Two months later, my wish was finally granted. I was set free! I was released. Eight freaking months of this ordeal were finally over. I had felt like a hostage for so long.

For Lindy, the day of her stroke was a time to reconnect with her faith. (As told with the assistance of her son, Chad).

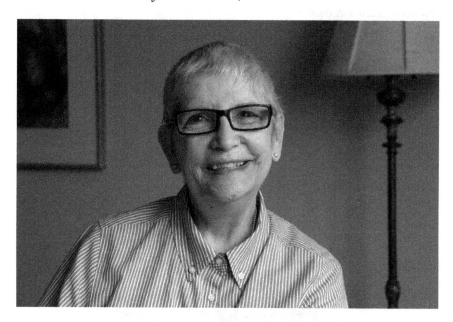

Brushes and colors, rather than words, have been her communication tools since childhood because they are intrinsic to her personality. This is truer now more than ever.

In 2000, Lindy suffered a massive stroke that paralyzed her right hand and left her with severe aphasia. She was in her 50s. Lindy is a painter, a Buddhist, and has a loving family, who is very involved with her care. She is very motivated and enthusiastically participates in all the aphasia program classes, but especially likes the art sessions. After a strenuous rehabilitation, Lindy picked up her brush again, this time with her left hand. The results have been astounding. Watching her style adapt, evolve and re-invent is inspiring. She credits her Buddhism with keeping her in a peaceful and positive state of mind.

Lindy trained at San Jose State College. She has shown in one-woman and group exhibitions in Los Angeles, San Francisco, Santa Rosa, London, and Scotland. Lindy has received private and corporate commissions in the United States, London, and Thailand. She works from her imagination and daily experience, portraying many colorful characters from dancers and jugglers, to her *Blind Detective* series, including his faithful companion.

Lindy currently lives in Pompton Plains, New Jersey. More information and artwork can be found at www.lindysart.com and www.strokebrush.com.

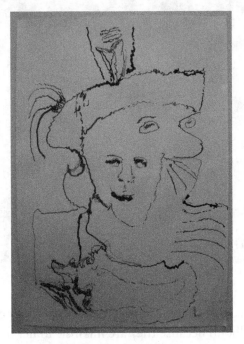

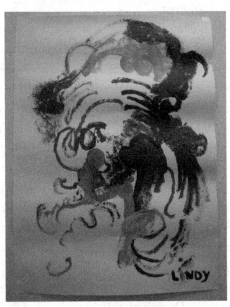

For Lee, his stroke was a life-changer, but not a life-ender. (Lee's story is told through the perspective of Yvonne Honigsberg.)

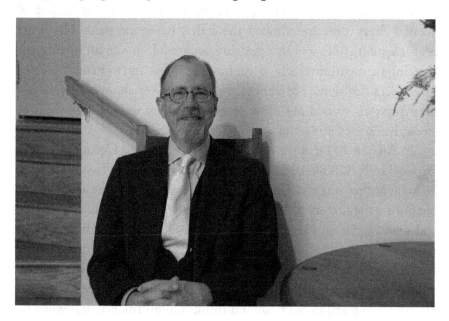

I first met Lee in a literature group at Metropolitan Communication Associates (MCA), an aphasia program affectionately known as Mona's program. Lee looks a bit like Freud, or an artist or writer, with round-rimmed glasses a la James Joyce. He's often dressed in a vest and tie, befitting an old-fashioned gentlemen. (This is not typical attire of the groups' clients!) Rather than being pretentious with so studied a look, I could quickly see he was genuine, unassuming, and modest.

Lee is relied on by many as a cultural reference. When the group comes across an esoteric word that baffles them, they turn to Lee, who infallibly always knows the meaning. He may not have the right words at the moment, often searching, grappling for words, but he often tries two or three times to get his meaning across. If the group doesn't get it the first time, he writes letters or words with his hands or writes a key word on a scrap of paper. Sometimes it requires guessing what he means, but he doesn't give up easily and perseveres. He usually gets his point across and makes himself understood.

Lee is proud of his family lineage, which can be traced back to the

1600s to one of the first settlers in America. He is related to President Tyler, who, ironically, died from a stroke.

Flashback to 2003. For several weeks, Lee was getting out of breath. Every time he climbed the stairs, he would pant. His heart beat irregularly. He was in a pressure cooker job in a small investment banking firm with pressure to get more business and to make the right investment decisions. He went to the doctor to see about his stress, but his symptoms turned out to be something more serious than signs of stress; he needed an operation.

In August 2004, at the age of 51, he went in for a Coronary Artery Bypass Graft (CABG), but the procedure didn't work. Two years later, he had another surgery. This time, it was successful as far as his heart, but during the surgery he had a stroke. He awoke to right-sided paralysis and severe aphasia. He could read, but suddenly he couldn't speak or write. Over time, he learned to say a few words, but they wouldn't be the right words. He couldn't name names or objects or put words in an order that made sense. For the first time ever, numbers were a problem. He could do math in his head and think in high finance, but when he tried to say numbers, he couldn't get it right.

He recovered from hemiparesis within six months, although he still has numbness on his right side. The aphasia is another story.

When Lee is asked about how aphasia effects him, he says, "Everything." It is the single biggest problem that effects everything he does that requires speaking or writing: shopping, asking for things, asking for directions, giving directions, asking and answering questions, making comments. I can see why he says "everything." When I ask him what helps with his aphasia, what aspects of therapy are effective, he says, "Everything. One-on-one helps the most." For instance, he lights up when talking about cutting edge restaurants and cooking gourmet dishes, and he gets to talk about this subject with his speech therapist.

When Lee had his stroke, he was knee-deep in his third career as an investment banker. He seemed too mild-mannered for a shark tank career, so I wasn't surprised to learn that he had two very different careers before that. At first he worked as an artist, a painter and photographer, then as an architect, working his way up to manager of the firm. Then Lee went back to school for an Executive MBA Program at NYU. Upon completing the graduate program, he began working as investment banker.

After his stroke, faced with the prospect of finding meaningful work, Lee decided to go into the antiques business. He opened up a French antiques gallery in Manhattan. Filled with early twentieth century antiques and fabrics from the Far East and an atelier, Bermingham & Co. was born. The premise was that the employees would handle speaking to customers, and Lee would take care of the business end, handling the financials. This, however, proved to be difficult with aphasia affecting his ability to write and say numbers. It was disappointing to realize that recovery was slow, but Lee knew that he still had business, investing, and artistic sensibilities, so he focused on making decisions on the selections of the antique pieces. He and his partners came up with creative ways to help the business survive and thrive during a time filled with economic struggles for the industry at-large.

Lee loves to cook. Sometimes his dishes are complex and artsy. Having a photography background, he often takes out his camera phone and shows pictures of gourmet dishes he has made: asparagus and roasted tomatoes, scallop and shrimp risotto, marrow bones displayed decoratively, laid out like a portrait or a still life painting. They are impressive to look at. Sometimes he comes up with the names of the food items easily. Other times, he can't recall or can't be easily understood, but this is getting better all the time.

Together with two close friends (who are also his business partners), Lee bought a sprawling property in Bucks County, Pennsylvania. It was a farm complete with a donkey and chickens. The three of them want to turn the barn into a warehouse for the antiques, while Lee wants to turn the chicken coop into a 3,800 square feet dream house. (The donkey is staying, thank you very much.)

Lee doesn't hesitate to show pictures of the property on his phone and draws rough sketches of his dream house on napkins. He has shown me a professional drawn-to-scale draft of the proposed house. He is looking forward to and working hard on building this dream house, which is his personal architectural challenge and labor of love. It will take more than three years to construct, but he hopes the result will be a gem he'll enjoy for years to come.

Lee loves to tango dance, with its sinuous lines and impassioned music, but after the stroke, he has more challenges. In tango and related dances, the male dancer gives signals to his dance partner to turn, but Lee couldn't tell how hard or soft he was pushing until a dance partner got upset with him for using more force than needed. He wasn't giving the right signals due to numbness in his right hand. He was dismayed and apologetic, but decided not to sit by the sidelines and quit. He still takes tango lessons trying to get the pressure right. In fact, during The Moth storytelling workshop, Lee told his story about his love of dancing Tango, even post-stroke. He finished with the line, "If you can tango, you can do anything." (See Chapter 5 to read Lee's story.)

For Yvonne, the day of her stroke on February 21, 2009 began as nothing more than a turn on the treadmill.

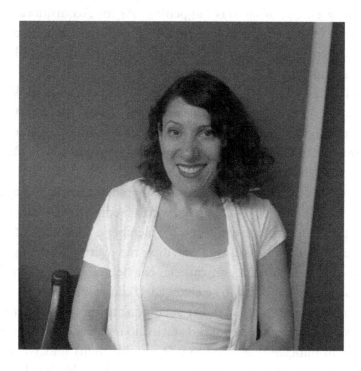

I had just hopped on the treadmill and was increasing the incline when I spotted the brand-new, sleek TVs suspended from the ceilings. I started to *ooo* and *ahh* and tried to comment on the sparkling new TVs to the person running next to me, but my voice came out slurred and garbled, like a drunkard. Suddenly, I felt wobbly and dizzy. Everything seemed to be in slow motion—my body droopy, not obeying my muscles. In seconds, I managed to jump off the treadmill before stumbling to the ground, the treadmill still whirring.

A woman in the gym shrieked, "Oh my God! Oh my God! Are you okay?" I tried to speak, but no words came out, like in a bad dream when you open your mouth and try to scream, but don't make a sound. I heard a woman speaking on the phone in a frenzied, hysterical voice. Another woman told me to just breathe, everything would be okay, help was on the way. One of the women held my hand and said, "Can you hear me? Okay, if you can hear me, just nod." I couldn't nod. Then she said, "Okay, if you can hear me, just blink." Tears started teeming out of my eyes as I lay on the gym floor, face up.

I knew exactly what was happening. As an Acquisitions Editor in Clinical Medicine, I had just commissioned a neurologist to write a book called *Acute Stroke Care*, and the symptoms fit the bill; *I* was having a stroke myself.

I was in a coma for three weeks in the ICU at the hospital. When I came to, my right arm couldn't move, my left "good" arm was strapped to the bed, and my right leg was in a royal blue splint, immobile. Most alarming of all, I couldn't speak a single word—not even a "Yes," or "No," or "What happened?"

Unable to communicate in words, I was rendered infant-like again—literally speechless, helpless, even fed with a feeding tube. Being unable to speak was *more* than frustrating. I remember a time, for instance, a nurse's aide in the hospital was watching me overnight, sitting at my bedside. Around 9:00 p.m., my catheter bag became full, and she didn't even look to see that it had to be changed. (I didn't know why I couldn't pee at the time, only that I couldn't.) I couldn't speak at all, so I used the only arsenal I had at my disposal: I started to moan and roll over in bed restlessly to indicate that I had to urinate. She didn't understand, just kept putting her finger to her lips and whispering, "Shh, Shhh, Shhh," to calm me down. I started moaning loudly, pleadingly, and then angrily because I had to empty my bladder urgently. Still she didn't understand. The one hand that I could have used was strapped to the bed (so as not to pull my tubes out once again), and I couldn't even gesture to tell her what I needed. Instead of changing my bag, she just kept offering me a drink of water, which was the last thing I needed! The urgent need to go to the bathroom went on for 10 excruciating hours. Relief finally came when the morning nurse came on duty.

After a month at the hospital, I was transferred to inpatient rehabilitation for six weeks more, went home, and began my journey through the many trials and tribulations, as well as a few triumphs, of rehabilitation. I had a year and a half of intense occupational, physical, and speech therapy, and some cognitive therapy.

Physical therapy was very frustrating for me because no matter how I tried—and I did try through countless exercises like electrostimulation, mirror therapy, etc.—I couldn't make my arm or hand work for the life of me. If I tried to open my hand and extend my fingers, it would make the opposite movement and recoil into a fist. I ended up feeling tearful and defeated many times.

The one thing I succeeded in improving was my speech, thanks to a bunch of tireless and encouraging speech therapists. I turned my attention to the things I could do better, like writing a blog, creating comedy events with a friend, storytelling, volunteering, and reading aloud creative pieces that I had written. It gave me something hopeful and positive in my life. I was back in the game again.

During the first three months after the stroke, I felt unbelievably free of self-consciousness. I didn't have to do anything to impress anyone. I could be cranky and let the world know about it. I grimaced without caring what I looked like, filterless, whether for better or for worse. One time, my friend visited me in the rehab hospital. She started to cry because the doctors said I couldn't walk yet, and maybe never would. I pulled the covers off of me, hopped out of my hospital bed, and demonstrated how, yes, I could indeed walk around! I had this fight in me to make it back from the brink, to grow, to experience, to stretch myself, to shrink back when it hurt, to get mad at therapists who wanted to stretch out my hands, to try again, to demonstrate what I could do. Never say never. Every act was met by encouragement. My sister, friends, nurses, and therapists were watching out for my safety, and, in my uninhibited state, I was daring and fearless.

I felt inexplicable, loving, empathic feelings for everyone around me. One nurse's aide that was caring for me, again on the overnight shift, told me about her village back in Kenya: how the people were so grateful for every shred of clothing and food that they got, how they celebrated things and acts of kindness. I teared up and committed then to donate tons of clothing to her village after I got out. I tried to dance a jig right there in my hospital gown. She laughed and shooed me back to bed.

Some friends said that it is because of my spirit and will and strength that I have gotten as far as I have. I take exception to that. I could have done more. There were a lot of extremely low times. I spent so much time in the dank basement of my dreams. Fear, anxiety, and self-loathing overtook me when I realized my arm and hand weren't coming back, that I would never talk normally again, never walk without a limp, never run.

I recently had an incident that serves as an analogy for my stroke experience. I decided to clean my computer and saturated the keyboard with Windex. Bad move. From then on, every time I tried to type certain letters, I got nothing but a blank screen. No matter what I did, it wouldn't respond. The keyboard looked fine, but it did not work right. When I'm sitting down and silent, I look fine, like there's nothing wrong with me. When I stand up and walk, in motion everyone can see that I can't use my right arm and hand and that I have a limp. When I try to speak, I'm outed as having trouble talking. "S's" become "Sh's," "single" becomes "shingle," "spell" becomes "smell," and so forth, courtesy of the bloodbath on my brain's left frontal lobe. I am like the computer screen trying to reboot.

There are many frustrating aspects of aphasia. The other day, for instance, I was telling a friend about a funny incident. I said, "I took food from Robert's plate...uh, uh, um." Stop here, an awkward pause. I search my brain's computer. "Seriously?" *No*, I say inside my head. "Sirly?" *No, that's not it.* "Secretly?" *Getting closer.* That will do, but it's not the exact word I want. "Surreptitiously!!" *Bingo!* That strikes the right chord.

My computer brain gets jammed, locked, frozen like my laptop's broken keys. The mouse gets...*uh, um, what do you call the pointed arrow thingamajig on the screen?* It is locked, frozen. Sometimes it gets lost altogether and disappears from the screen. Hey... *Cursor! Bingo again.* I love when I remember words. *Reboot.* It's like a jigsaw puzzle; only the exact pieces fit.

My speech is slowed down by the cognitive overload of searching for the right word. When I find it or something close to it, then I have to say it in the right order, with proper grammar and correct pronunciation. I have relatively mild aphasia, dysarthria, and apraxia, but the many "senior moments," and the effort it takes to over-enunciate my words to be understandable, makes speech much more effortful and taxing. It's tempting to not speak up at all sometimes, but to participate in conversations, to express, to understand, and be understood is worth the fight.

Twain said, "The difference between the almost right word and the right word is the difference between lightening and the lightning bolt." He wasn't thinking about aphasia, but it fits well. Often I have to settle for a "close enough" word and a "good enough" pronunciation, but sometimes I get the lightning bolt—and it soars through the air.

"The Petal"

Surprised by a single bright red rose petal, I thought it was something of a metaphor for what happened to me—my hemorrhagic stroke came out of nowhere, like an illusion, a terrifying, peculiar dream. After I got out of the hospital, I was full of new life and inspiration, a somewhat magical time for me because I had survived, albeit with other, major struggles due to my brain blood burst, including aphasia. Writing this poem connected me to my "old voice," not my slurred, struggling voice.

There it was, like a magic trick
for me

There wasn't a rose in sight,
but it lay there shining up
from the concrete slab of
sidewalk,
like an invitation, a tease—a
petal.

The two objects revealing their
souls,
One gritty, matte, pedestrian
One ethereal, almost levitating,
The color of blood—the real
Color in its surprising burst or trickle
of warm color, not the deeper
color when it dries.

Delicate as skin,
The expanse of rich velvet
A little white spot where

it broke off the stem
A grand carpet for an ant

If I bent down to retrieve it
It would disappear, a figment
Like a cat chasing a light
reflected on the floor

Rich red running through
deep crannies and crevices
encased inside my skull, too.

Inside the arteries and veins
There lay globules of fat,
a gray hose tangled up tightly
that I could never touch or see
with my own senses

I would have to take it for
granted

Take on faith

That my brain looked the same
And acted the same
As everybody else's

Except when it didn't.

    —Yvonne Honigsberg

For Tamar, her Traumatic Brain Injury (TBI) may have altered her life, but it didn't alter her character. Tamar has been working extremely hard with cognitive work to address her decline in processing information, response time, topic maintenance, and verbal conciseness.

Having been a nurse, I understand that people get wrapped up in "going through the motions," but I want to remind medical professionals that the patients should not be treated as "labels." It is sometimes hard to see that each patient is an individual, but you have to realize at all times that people in comas are not "sacks of potatoes." We still have feelings. I had both positive and negative experiences through my journey to recovery.

As I want to end my story on a positive note, I'll share with you the negative nuances of my TBI first. They, the medical staff, made me feel invisible: The first thing I remember when I was in the coma was being taken to get an MRI; they pushed me around like a "sack of potatoes." Another memory I had while I was still in the coma was hearing the nurses talk about me as if I was not even in the room. I had one nurse say to another nurse, "It's okay, you don't need to attend to Tamar. She's fine." What if I wasn't okay? They didn't even check to see. A small trait like empathy goes a long way for a patient in recovery. They lacked it. When I needed to go to the bathroom, no one ever came when I buzzed them. I leaned against the walls and pillars to get to the bathroom. I finally got there on my own and fell to the floor. I remember when the nurse came in, I was holding onto the toilet and the first thing the nurse said to me was, "Why are you hugging the toilet when you have such a cute husband?" They never even asked if I was okay. I was already experiencing so many emotions, ranging from anger to confusion. The last emotion I wanted to feel was crazy. The medical staff succeeded; they made me feel crazy. I remember that you could see a family of turkeys from outside my window. One day, I tried to walk to the window so I could see them. When the nurse asked what I was doing, I told her that I wanted to see the turkeys, and she treated me like I was a crazy person.

While others may have fallen into depression and given up, I was lucky in that this experience made me push harder. I felt that I had to fight to prove them wrong. However, not all experiences were bad, and the little, genuine kind acts that people did during my recovery made such a difference. Every smile and every kind word is hope to live.

My most memorable positive moment happened after critical care. I remember the nurse helping me to get dressed showed her beautiful kindness willingly. The nurse commented to me, "Look at all the new clothes you get to wear!" She made me feel excited about something, even if it was something small. Although I don't remember the nurse's face or her name, I can remember how the nurse made me feel: so very happy. In my physical therapy, the kind, reassuring, and encouraging sessions would always end with pointing out my achievements as well as a reminder to remember safety first. It made me feel that the physical therapist genuinely cared. My doctors would also always turn the negatives into positives, which helped me to never lose faith.

Eight years later, I still feel the warmth and encouragement that these people gave me. Not everyone is a fighter like me, and many can get discouraged; however, all that people in these situations need are small acts of kindness to remind them what they want to live for and hope for during the state that they are in.

My time with Mona and the Metropolitan Communications Association (MCA) further expanded the idea that a small act of kindness goes a long way. MCA is a family, a community, a support system, and a place to boost your confidence. This is a comfortable, open, caring environment. This place meets all my needs, both physically and emotionally.

Before coming to MCA, I was never satisfied. Being aware what you have lost, you want to get back to what you were. Here at MCA, everybody takes you for who you are; they are kind and accepting. You have others who can understand the situation you are in, and professionals that provide the empathy and support you need. I feel it is important to have a place that not only understands you, but where they encourage you, a place where you can grow. Living in a place like New York City, everyone outside looks at you like you're incomplete, but coming to a place like MCA you can start to believe in yourself. It is a safe zone that allows you to grow and begin to feel complete again.

For Avi, having a stroke did not mean putting his life on hold. It meant working harder to make that leap. (From the perspective of Yvonne Honigsberg.)

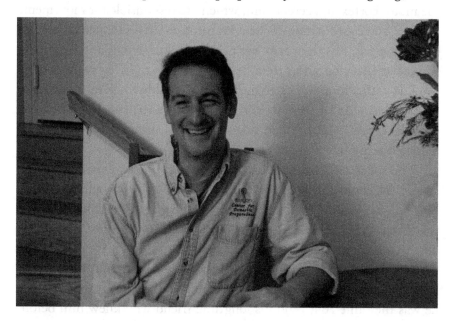

Avi had a stroke in 2007, when he was 35. His aphasia affects his speaking and writing, but not reading. He also has difficulty with word searching and grammar. Avi loves to gather people together (those disabled and their loved ones) for outdoor sports, museum-going, and other activities. He is the founder of New York Outdoor Club and has a penchant for extreme sports, including skydiving and scuba diving. He is also a tireless advocate for aphasia and speaks to many speech therapy classrooms and other audiences. Avi helps train EMTs and other affiliated health professionals in recognizing and working with people who have aphasia. He participates in countless activities, including acting in plays through an aphasia group and traveling to Israel and the Caribbean. He hopes to go back to medical school and become a doctor, specializing in emergency medicine.

Avi is infectiously gregarious. He was a certified paramedic who loved helping people in urgent medical crises, and in his spare time he could be seen skydiving out of planes, rock climbing, and snowboarding. He was about to start medical school to become an ER doctor when he opted to have heart surgery to get it "out of the way" before school. During surgery he had a stroke that damaged the Broca's and Wernicke's regions of the brain, which involve speech, and the motor cortex and cerebellum, which are responsible for movement, balance, and coordination. When Avi came out of his induced coma, he couldn't speak. His right arm was paralyzed and floppy, and like many stroke patients who suffer from hemiparesis, his right leg swung out to the side with a limp. Once gregarious, Avi couldn't talk to friends and family, he couldn't do his job, and he couldn't participate in his beloved outdoor sports. His life had taken a radical, unexpected twist that rendered him mute and physically disabled.

The most difficult part was his aphasia. For two years after his stroke, Avi could only say one word—Michael. When people asked him how he was (Was he hungry? Did he want to go outside?), his response was always Michael, like a broken record stuck in a groove. He claims now that he doesn't know who Michael was.

His career dreams dashed and his future foggy, Avi managed to keep up a brave face. "From the moment he woke up in the hospital, he was the same Avi," said his longtime friend who knew him before his stroke. "Even though he couldn't speak, Avi was exactly the same person, warm and charming! You could tell he had the same friendliness and spirit that he had before his stroke."

Immediately after the stroke, Avi experienced depression for the first time in his life, but he didn't give up. Eventually he rallied and sought many different treatments—the usual course of post-stroke occupational, physical, and speech therapies. Over time, he threw into the mix acupuncture, Feldenkrais water therapy, and Tai Chi, among others. He participated in rehabilitation research studies for aphasia and hemiparesis and helped test robotic devices.

In the process, he met world-renowned doctors, nurses, therapists, and stroke/TBI survivors. His enthusiasm, friendliness, and spirit made an impression on many of them, and quite a few of whom became his friends.

I met Avi the first time I dug up my courage to attend our support group. I'd had a devastating stroke only the year before, and I was going through a rough patch. When I walked into the room, a young man grinned at me openly and welcomingly. After he saw that I had difficulty speaking, he approached me, motioned to his chest, and said,

"Avi" and "Speech. Come! Mona. Come! Awesome." No sooner did I perk up and show interest, then he whipped out his cell phone and generously gave me the phone number and address of his beloved speech and language pathologist Dr. Mona Greenfield.

It seems that Avi is everywhere. "There is a running joke in NYC stroke survivor circles that everybody knows Avi!" a physical therapist said. She thought of getting a T-shirt that says, "I know Avi Golden." "That's a testament to how widespread his outreach is to people with aphasia and disabled people in the New York City area," she added.

From the perspective of Mona Greenfield.

Throughout five years of working with Avi, he has persevered and worked on improving communication. In the beginning, Avi could only say one word and needed significant support to get his words out. Avi has always been very social and had a strong desire to read, listen, write, and speak about his thoughts, feelings, and ideas. Through his determination, he emails, reads, and discusses articles related to aphasia and disabilities and requests endless speech and language therapy with the hope of realizing his dreams and inspiring individuals with disabilities to do the same.

From the perspective of Ellayne S. Ganzfried.

Avi is truly an extraordinary champion for aphasia advocacy! His contributions are making a difference to the entire aphasia community. He has taken what most would consider a tragedy and turned it into an opportunity to be a leader. It has been remarkable for me to see the progress Avi has made with his own communication skills as he educates others about aphasia. It has forced him to focus on his reading, writing, and oral presentation in the context of something meaningful to him— raising awareness of aphasia in the community and training health care professionals and emergency responders. This is truly an example of the Life Participation Approach to aphasia in action. He is unwavering in his commitment and tenacity to be heard. His enthusiasm, energy, and can-do attitude are contagious. It has been my pleasure to have him support the National Aphasia Association (NAA) and to work together to raise awareness of aphasia.

For D'Angelo, a man of many talents, his stroke was an unexpected obstacle that he continues to overcome with a stellar positive attitude.

On Easter Sunday 2011, I went out to a friend's birthday dinner at The Olive Garden, and then we went to another party. I started feeling funny, unstable; I passed out and the rest is history.

I woke up three weeks later in the hospital, and I couldn't recognize anybody that was present. I couldn't speak or write, I couldn't spell, I couldn't pronounce any words at all. I was 50 lbs lighter, barely recognizing things as before. I kept staring at myself in the mirror because while I was in the coma, I saw myself through different eyes.

Then I was told that I had had a stroke! I wasn't really surprised to hear it, because I had already endured two strokes prior to this. I was diagnosed as having aphasia, and it would change my whole life.

I stayed in the hospital seven more days. I discovered that I stuttered now. I never stuttered before. I had to relearn putting on clothes, washing up, reading, writing. I virtually had to start my life over.

In the mornings, I would go to occupational therapy with my occupational therapist, and in the afternoon, I would attend sessions with my speech-language pathologist (SLP). She was my first SLP— she was really good—then I got another one, then another one, then another one, etc., etc. Nonetheless, I kept on learning. (Later on, I found out the SLP's were actually students studying speech.)

Then my occupational therapist got me to attend the Young Stroke Survivor's Support Group, and it exposed me to a whole bunch of people who were going through the same thing I was going through. I found another group founded by a stroke survivor. He is a stroke survivor who also uses Melodic Intonation Therapy (MIT). I still went to the hospital everyday for the next year and half. I broke the record of patients who kept on coming.

Early on after the stroke, I traveled to Portland, Oregon, Hollywood and Las Vegas, but as soon as I got back, my life started falling apart. I started having problems in my relationship. I couldn't keep up with paying the rent for the studio. I couldn't read or write, and I could barely talk. After thinking about it for a while, I wasn't really doing any music and my relationship was on the outs. I decided to let them both go and focus on the problem at hand—aphasia!

After taking two and half months off, I went to an event hosted by the National Aphasia Association, and I met Avi, a stroke survivor and advocate for getting the word out about aphasia. So, I teamed up with him because by that time I wanted to let people know about aphasia. He had teams of people that would go to colleges, universities, and speech clinics and talk about aphasia. It was Avi, Yvonne, Rob, a couple of others and now me. I'm really proud of that. It's a beautiful thing.

I've seen a lot of changes in my fellow aphasic colleagues, as well as myself. We are all getting better! Not all at once, but we are taking gradual strides towards the top. We're doing it.

Now, I don't think about music at all. I still have all my equipment, just in case I get that musical bug back. I bought a camera just before the trip, and now I take pictures and edit them. I also work out a lot because going to the gym helps me stay focused. It gives me another goal to shoot for.

For almost a year now, Avi has wanted me to join his SLP, Mona Greenfield. I finally met with her one day after a presentation. We talked, it was a fit, and we started right away. I met her incredible clinicians, SLPs, social workers, and students. My SLP, a student, and the social worker helped me with both strategies and real life situations. The SLP and student always teased me about recording myself, to let me know how much better I've gotten. I'm kind of hard on myself.

Honestly, I didn't sign up for aphasia. It was something that came along with the stroke. It's really hard to live with, but we've got to do it. To my peers, hopefully this inspires you just as much as all of you have inspired me.

Lastly, I want to thank the hospital. They are going to close their doors for good this week. The stroke unit, occupational therapy, and speech department took such good care me.

Thank you,
    Angelo.

For Fran, a former dancer and teacher, a stroke was the beginning of allowing her fighting spirit to shine through.

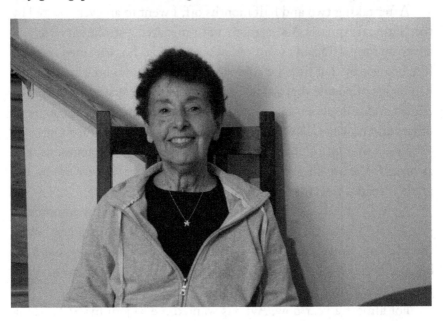

I was in the middle of doing something, when I fell and couldn't get up. That's the day that I had my stroke. I waited until my mother and father came home, and when they saw me, they were in shock. But I couldn't say anything. At twenty-four years old, there was nothing I could say. I was coughing, coughing, coughing; I could barely breathe.

At the hospital, they had to put me in a private room because I kept coughing. I remember the doctors coming in and saying, "Francine you had a stroke." Again, I couldn't say anything. It was miserable. Death flashed before me. My mind knew what was wrong, but I couldn't express myself through words.

Later, I went right into surgery and had a tracheotomy performed to allow me to breathe without the use of my nose or mouth. The surgery ended, and I was in a coma. The doctors told my parents, "She may make it, and she may not," and my mom said, "She's my daughter, she'll make it." Mom was right. I did come out of the coma. I remember feeling out of breath and sitting up. All I could see was red, white, and blue.

I was in the hospital for about six months. It felt beautiful the day that I left. I remember that day; the doctor said to my parents, "Give her anything she wants." They did; they gave me everything I wanted, and that day all I wanted was Chinese food.

Over the next few months, I lost a lot of weight. I was only seventy pounds. I was a total mess and needed a lot of help during that time. My parents and my grandmother, who'd temporarily moved into our house, helped me tremendously. My family was very good to me.

I was home for a couple of weeks, and then I went into rehabilitation for speech. It was very hard to talk. In fact, five years passed, and I still couldn't speak. During that time, I lost my father and my grandmother. It was a difficult period in my life, but I was determined to get better. I would listen to music and try to say the lyrics, trying to get my speech back through music.

After four years, my mother said, "Talk already! Talk!" My mother was frustrated, and I got even more frustrated. It was terrible what she said, because I wanted to talk but couldn't.

After five years, thank God, I started talking again. I remember the first thing I said was, "Oh, shit!" That was no coincidence. Over the last several decades, my speech has gotten better and better. Today, after all that I've been through, I really feel like a winner.

For Rob, his strokes became a journey of reinventing and looking forward.

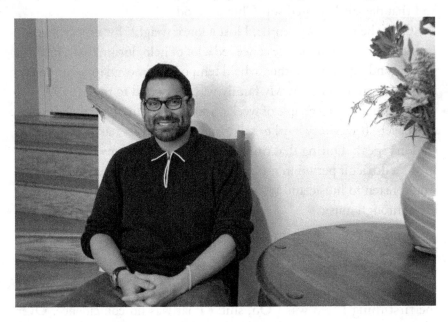

(Note: Rob had help writing his story down due to trouble with word finding, grammar, syntax, and overall writing, but that is getting better over time.)

In 2001, I had a job that I really liked. I made videos and films for a large, well-known advertising agency. Then, when I was 27, I had a stroke. Two years later, I had two consecutive strokes. The fourth stroke was in 2011.

After my third stroke, my aphasia returned and stuck. I couldn't talk to people at all at first. My family was amazing and really rose to the occasion. They all came together to help support me in this emotional journey. My sister came up from Florida to help me. I couldn't speak, so she had to help make doctors' appointments, cancel credit cards, apply for benefits, etc. She helped me immensely.

I began taking an ESL class, where I met my future wife, Nevin. She is from Turkey and wanted to learn English, so we were both taking an English learning class. Of course, she didn't know what the word aphasia meant, and I couldn't explain it because of the very fact that I had it. At first she thought that I was an Italian student trying to learn English, but eventually she understood. I am working hard to improve my aphasia by reading, books like *Game of Thrones*, while listening to audiotapes and going to Mona's program twice a week. At Mona's, I like one-on-one speech therapy best of all. I've noticed there's been improvement in my abilities to use numbers, like getting the date right and answering math questions.

I also go to the gym, doing a lot of cardio—the treadmill, bicycle, and StairMaster—and eating healthier food. My mother and wife are great cooks, so it's hard to resist their delicious food, but I succeed a lot more. I try to relax a lot more, to just enjoy things more in life and spend quality time with my family and my wife. I travelled with my wife to Turkey and stayed a couple of months. Talking to my mother and my wife helps with my aphasia, supporting the adage, "If you don't use it, you lose it."

A few years ago, I started a blog called "World of Aphasia." Why? Most people don't know that strokes can happen in younger people. Second of all, most people haven't even heard the word "aphasia," let alone know what it means. As is common with a lot of people with aphasia, word finding, spelling, and grammar are very difficult for me, making writing impossible for now, but I *can* copy and paste with the best of them. So I paste different articles on the subject to make people aware of what it is, and what's it like. Maybe it will enhance understanding, compassion, and patience.

Little by little, I am getting better. It helps to have structure and understanding in my life. I notice my math skills getting better through Mona's program. I used to spend a lot of time just thinking after my stroke. Now I do more. I know now that acting is better. I realize more and more that I can be captain of my own ship.

.... ▬▬▬▬▬▬▬▬▬▬▬▬▬▬▬▬▬

CHAPTER 7

A Helping Hand: Caregiver Stories
Home Health Care Attendants
Mona Greenfield, PhD, LCSW, CCC-SLP

Many people with aphasia need to rely on home health care attendants or aides for their daily care. For some, this care is in addition to the support of family caregivers, and for others the aide is their primary caregiver. These individuals are with the person with aphasia during the day and oftentimes for 24 hours, providing round-the-clock care.

Coordinating home care needs in general can be complicated and involves the interaction of many agencies. These issues are further compounded when the care is for a person with aphasia (PWA), due to the accompanying communication challenges. Assistance can be provided with activities of daily living, such as dressing, bathing, light cleaning, cooking, shopping, doing laundry, making appointments, and accompanying the person to appointments. Home health aides also can serve as companions and join the PWA for social outings.

We spoke to several aides to get their input. All of the aides indicated that they did not know anything about aphasia when they were hired. They also expressed that they did not receive specific training by any agency to understand aphasia or how to communicate with and care for an individual with aphasia. They acknowledged that they learned on the job from watching the therapists work with their clients. Through this experience they learned to slow down their speech, write words on paper, repeat information, and wait patiently for the PWA to get out their words. One aide said that she "never heard the word aphasia at her agency" and she "did not think that her agency knew what aphasia was."

Through the process of living, working, and observing therapy sessions with PWAs, many of the aides have learned how to better communicate with their clients and ultimately provide better care. Since the communication difficulties presented are different for each person with aphasia, a basic understanding of the comprehension and expressive communication processes, as well as strategies to enhance these skills, would be most helpful to attendants and aides assigned by agencies to work with these individuals.

A Stroke from a Caregiver's Point of View by Ina

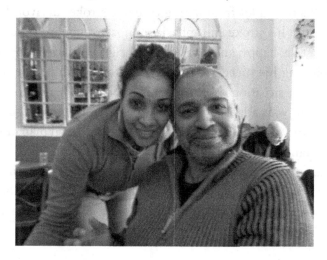

I am a caregiver, or Personal Care Attendant (PCA), for my godfather, who had a stroke in August 2010. Although I always knew people were affected by strokes, I guess I never gave thought that one day it would take over one of my loved ones. As Albert, my godfather, says, "A stroke is no joke." There is nothing to be taken lightly about a stroke. From the person who experiences the stroke to the family, the friends, and even the person's job, everything is turned upside-down by this disease.

When I first saw my godfather in the hospital, where he was for a total of eight months, I was completely paralyzed for a brief moment. I couldn't grasp how a person goes from verbal to non-verbal, from eating on his own to a feeding tube, etc. At that point, I realized that the stroke had completely consumed him, and my concern was, would he ever be the man I had once known? With the love, faith, and support of his wife/angel, he pulled through, and four years later, he is still improving each day.

Caring for someone on a daily basis is not as easy as it seems. Caregivers also get tired, stressed, anxious, and impatient at times.

With that said, I also have to admit that being a caregiver has completely humbled me. It has reminded me not to take the little things for granted, and I personally feel proud and satisfied with the work I do every day. Having a stroke is not a walk in the park, but being a caregiver isn't either. A stroke survivor and a caregiver work hand-in-hand as a team every day.

I have learned a lot from taking care of a stroke survivor. I also see how important his stroke and aphasia support groups are. These groups keep him active, happy, and distracted. The groups have many benefits, from improving his speech to surrounding him with people that have been in similar situations. A stroke survivor has to deal with living his life a different way, adapting on a daily basis. A caregiver also needs to embrace caring for someone and being their right-hand man or woman, their confidant, and their support.

Stroke survivors are to be admired, but I think oftentimes their caregivers don't get the credit we should. Good caregivers should not be taken for granted and should definitely have their stories told and listened to more often.

Founding of a Mother-Son Research and Development Team by Chad

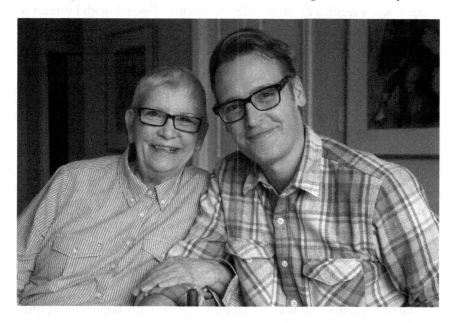

When my mother, Lindy, had her stroke, we both lived on opposite coasts—me in New York and her in northern California. I had to figure out my role as long-distance caregiver, doing what I could to support her partner. I handled some of her insurance logistics and was present for regular video chats and phone calls. As often as my work schedule would permit, I travelled across the country to provide her partner respite from the demands of being my mom's primary caregiver and language partner. I enjoyed these visits to her small ranch house in Sebastopol, California. Her house was surrounded by pine trees and was bounded by a small stream, a stark contrast to the bang and clatter of New York City life.

My mom, an accomplished artist before her stroke, worked quietly on a painting using her left hand, while I tapped away on my computer, keeping work obligations at bay. Aside from the click of my keyboard and the quiet scratching of my mother's pencil, the room was particularly quiet that afternoon. Medications were up to date. Physical and speech therapy obligations had been met. It was a moment to relish, mother-and-son time together, each of us engaged in our own personal work.

But there was something about the quiet that was also disconcerting.

I noticed that the phone didn't ring as much as it had during previous visits. Friends seemed to check in less frequently. Even though I was away from home, I was in close contact with my wife and kids and siblings via email and text messages. Like a lot of people, my communication habits had shifted away from the telephone into other forms of communication, the very modes of communication that were impossible for my mom to use. At first, I thought this was just a generational thing, which to a certain extent was likely true. But my mom's friends were also using the phone less frequently. They too were gravitating to text, email, and social networks to stay in touch.

The stroke left Mom with severe aphasia that made keyboards pretty much impossible for her to use. We had made some attempts to get her to assemble words, but it was clear that this wasn't going to work out. I might as well have been asking her to type a message in a foreign language. The ubiquitous keyboard was confusing, cluttered, and nonsensical to her aphasic brain.

Mom's friends still wanted to be in touch with her and certainly sent her emails, which often sat unread for days and sometimes weeks until a busy caregiver could log in, read them to her, and sometimes assist her with a reply. The more honest of her friends confessed, with some overt sense of guilt, that they found talking on the phone with her to be challenging; conversations were too one-sided, and they often had to have the context to tease out even the slightest detail of Mom's day. Many friends simply faded away. I learned later that this is a very common experience for people who have been through a debilitating event. Their friends can't handle the change, whether it's due to a fear of their own mortality or simply a lack of compassion. People often can't make the connection between who someone once was and who they are after a stroke. Certainly, Mom made many new friends along the way, who were supportive and caring and who more than made up for the notable absentees. Really, you might want to think about that further. Many people with aphasia feel hurt by the loss of some friends that they had before their strokes/injuries who may find it difficult to maintain their relationships after the person acquires aphasia.

By 2011, phone calls from friends were few and far between. People had really migrated to text, email, and especially Facebook as primary modes of updating, sharing, and communicating with the people they care about, and it really hit home for Mom. A worldwide communication revolution was happening all around her with new modes of communication being created regularly, yet Mom was unable to benefit from any of it. It was like being shut out of a huge gabfest. Email and texts were out of the question. Simply logging in to websites was a challenge rife with frustration. The busy interface of Facebook, with so much going on, was an enigma.

Mom had lived a cosmopolitan and international life. She has a daughter in Brighton, England and friends in Thailand and Connecticut and everywhere in between. Her inability to independently communicate electronically hindered her sense of connection to those that she loved. My mom is an unusually social person, who enjoys the company of so many different kinds of people, and I watched her retreat into herself. She became discouraged by the slow progress of her speech therapy. While she was simply overjoyed when her friends visited or phoned her, too many days were quiet and lonely.

I desperately wanted her to feel more connected to all the far-flung friends and loved ones. As a remote caregiver, I wanted to easily share photos and little anecdotes throughout my day as easily as sending a text message. But the barriers were tremendous. I knew there must be a way to bridge this accessibility gap. So, I tinkered with inventions, prototyped and broke some stuff, then prototyped some more. We formed a kind of mother-son research and development team as I explored high-tech and low-tech solutions for aiding our communication. Along the way, I created a gestural-based interface using a sensor that allowed her to send her first unassisted email. The message was simple, but she composed it using a visual dashboard. I played with physical interfaces with dials and buttons. Then, I got her an iPad as soon as they came out and created a simple, icon-based, messaging tool. She played with this for months and helped refine it before we made it available to other people in the form of Tapgram, a web-based application that aims to make social sharing as simple as possible. It's a social network simplified and stripped to the bare minimum of functionality.

Mom uses it to share her feelings, updating over fifty friends about what's going on in her day. She can look at pictures of her grandchildren from the other side of the globe and post picture replies. She can message a friend that she is thinking about them and that she wants to hear from them. She uses is several times a day, every day.

Notably, something else happened to Mom in the course of using Tapgram. Since using it, she has also had the most noticeable improvement in her speech and attitude. While this can be attributed to a variety of factors (Tapgram has certainly made her feel more connected and less isolated), she has also gained social media fluency.

After several weeks of using Tapgram, I noticed activity on her Facebook feed. She was "liking" things more and sharing things. In one sense this was a little bit disheartening. Having spent a lot of time and energy on Tapgram, did Mom even need it anymore? If Mom had been able to easily use Facebook, I might not have perceived the need for something more accessible, cleaner, and easier to use. But something really exciting happened, she started to attempt to type messages. I didn't prompt her. Honestly, I had given up on keyboards for her years earlier. It just seemed so insurmountable. For the first time in twelve years, Mom attempted, with some success, to type out messages. She had gone from being a complete social media non-participant to having working proficiency of Facebook and the keyboard. Interestingly, I noticed that her notebooks, usually filled with pictures started to include some words—phrases that she had seen through Facebook on her friend's feeds, written repeatedly as practice.

In addition to her use of the keyboard and attempts at writing words by hand, her vocabulary and enunciation underwent a leap of improvement. After years of celebrating the smallest increments of improvement, we found that she was finding new phrases, composing sentences, and attempting to tell more complex stories. Thirteen years after her stroke, there was renewed hope that there were still so many meaningful milestones to accomplish.

Certainly there are many factors for improvement in a stroke survivor. She has been actively dedicated and consistent with her speech therapy. She has moved closer to her grandkids and sees them more often. I know that Tapgram has also helped her, not just because of the technology that allows her to independently send messages—that would be quite a claim to make—but because it was born of a collaboration rooted in caring. That is where all the impact is, in caregiving. We are both grateful that our collaboration has helped thousands of others communicate with each other. Some of our users are stroke survivors, others are autistic. Tapgram has been used in a multi-modal schoolroom of hearing-impaired students, and many of Tapgram's users are "regularly" abled people who just appreciate its simplicity.

My Journey with Lewis by Helen

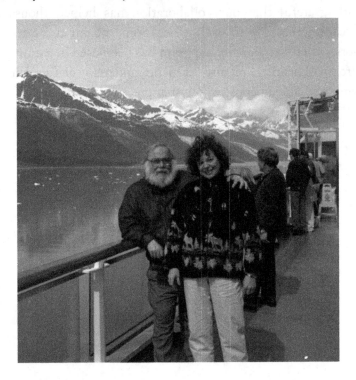

After my husband's stroke, I felt a tremendous responsibility, as though I held Lewis' life in my hands. I was terrified of doing the wrong thing, making a mistake. I felt like I was holding a soft chick with a fluttering heartbeat. Warmth, comfort, recovery, it was all up to me. Lew lay with his head wrapped in bandages, a hole in his throat to help him breathe, a hole in his stomach to help him take nutrition. At the time, he was quite heavy. I remember times, pitying the hospital staff, I would help to turn him. And later, pitying his inability to adjust himself on the bed, I would put his arm around my neck and lift him myself.

Aphasia. Before Lewis' stroke, I had simply never heard of it. Indeed, though I knew that stroke was the third major cause of death in this country, I had never met anyone who was living with a stroke. For many who suffer stroke, particularly with aphasia, life becomes increasingly isolated, friends falling by the wayside as they either can't or won't take the time to communicate with an aphasic or to re-examine what their friendship is about. With aphasia, relationships change. A friendship that is all about easy, intimate communication can no longer be that. Not because the aphasic has become unsympathetic or distant, but because conversation, the gateway to emotion, to connection, is broken, damaged, and sometimes completely gone.

One of the qualities that attracted me to Lewis when we first met was his ability to sustain long-held, close friendships with both men and women. I knew that his friends looked to him for a sympathetic ear and a keen mind. He was generous with his time, his love, and his money. People just naturally gravitated to him for advice, counsel, and support, and that core group, who he had known for decades, stuck with him. They came to see him at the brain injury rehab center that he went to for eight months. They sat and listened to him and tried to understand what he was thinking as he repeatedly responded, "Here, here." When he came home, most of them continued to come and see him, to spend time in mostly one-sided conversation, to celebrate his birthday. And they came to his funeral.

We were very lucky that way. I have heard numerous stories of friends, even family, falling by the wayside. At first, I would judge these people very harshly, after seven years, not so much. I have become much more humble about judging someone until I have been in their skin.

With aphasia, the caregiver is often placed in the role of translator. Even though I could sometimes spend twenty minutes trying to understand what Lewis wanted for lunch, people just naturally assumed that I understood everything that was on his mind. When one or two people would visit, I would subtly try to train them to communicate directly with Lewis, not through me. As they looked at me, rather than him, I would turn my head to Lewis, hoping that the others would naturally mimic me and look at him as well. Sometimes this worked, other times they remained locked on me, hoping that I held the key to Lewis' thoughts.

He was tremendously frustrated by this, and if we were speaking to a doctor or attorney, he would touch that person's arm and then point to himself, saying, "Me, me." The doctor, abashed, would look at Lewis for a few minutes and then gradually drift toward looking at me again. I loved that Lewis would insist that they look at him. He didn't let go until the person fully understood that it was he, Lewis, that was to be reckoned with.

He insisted with doctors, nurses, aides, therapists, and later, nursing home staff, that he was an individual and not just the patient or the resident. He was endearing, enraging, and charming. No one ever forgot him. As in his pre-stroke life, Lewis made his mark wherever he went, his strength of character and personality besting the aphasia that threatened to turn him into another cog in the wheel of the system.

Socially, one-on-ones weren't bad, but if we sometimes went out with a group of friends, especially to a noisy restaurant, Lewis was completely cut out of the conversation. None of this was malicious, but he simply couldn't process the cacophony, and people in a group tend to cross-talk, which is anathema to aphasics. This was devastating to both of us, and often we would leave the restaurant—me almost in tears, Lewis with his fist balled up in frustration. Over the years, we would be invited to events or dinners, and I would be tempted to either not tell him about it or discourage him from going. I just couldn't take the frustration and pressure. But I would never do it. I knew how much it meant to Lewis to feel connected, part of the world with a life bigger than his limitations. So, we went. Afterwards, we would commiserate with each other, but we went.

When we found out about a combination therapy/conversation group that met on Saturday mornings, it was as though we had discovered an underground community known only to us. We first started going about a year after Lewis' stroke, and I will never forget our delight in meeting this wonderful group of people struggling to speak, enjoying each other's company, and so willing to listen to Lewis' repeated "Here, here."

At around the same time, Lewis began attending a therapy program conducted by Dr. Mona Greenfield and speech therapists in training. Mona and her staff were wonderful in working individually with the patients, and, at least in Lewis' case, tailoring their therapeutic techniques to his skills and strengths. But the goal of the program, what set it apart from other speech therapy programs, was the group sessions with patients conversing, singing, discussing current events, and talking about different cultures. Oh how Lewis loved this. Being naturally curious and a flirt, he loved meeting the students who had come to the program from Russia, India, Brazil, and numerous other countries. He always had adored travel and managed to make friends wherever he went. Vicariously, through the tales of the students, he could "travel" once again.

While I am a tenacious, stubborn person, who finds it hard to take no for an answer, I simply didn't know how to navigate the thicket of federal and state rules, of bureaucratic layers, and of institutional blockheadedness that confronts the family of a catastrophically ill person. I feel very fortunate to have been helped in those beginning stages by the son of a family friend, who so fortuitously happened to be an eldercare lawyer.

He figuratively and literally held my hand in those first months, accompanying me to the Human Resources Administration to begin the process of applying for Medicaid. As I became increasingly acquainted with the system, I understood how twisted the system is, forcing loving, loyal couples into the position of considering "Medicaid Divorce" to preserve benefits.

In this situation, divorce becomes a planning tool that helps reduce the overall amount of assets a couple has to their name, thereby helping each spouse qualify for Medicaid without losing their entire life savings or investment properties.

I became shameless in asking for help. This went against the way I had been brought up, to regard asking for help as exposing vulnerability. I had thought that if you expose vulnerability, then others will see you as weak. I found the opposite to be true. I think that people wondered at my ability to get help, from institutions, bureaucracies, and individuals. I didn't take a "no" personally and immediately went on to the next person or spoke to a supervisor, whatever it took.

I often think of other caregivers I met through the years, perhaps not as stubborn or persistent as I, or perhaps just too tired. How many opportunities for new therapies or programs had they missed because no one had reached out to them, or because the information was not always easy to access?

Finally, there is no finally. Lewis died in the summer of 2014. Perhaps it is just too early to reflect with any kind of objectivity, except to say that aphasics and those who love them are caught in a terrible trap. Recently, I have begun to recapture memories of Lewis before his stroke, before everything changed. It is a blessing and a curse to remember.

A Different Life By Janice

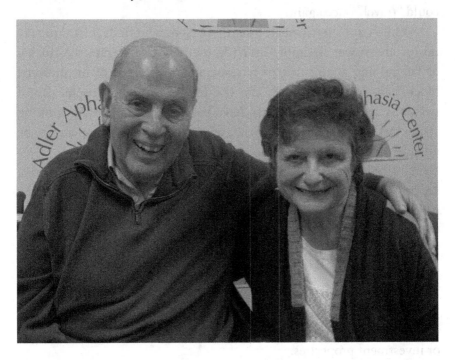

My husband Charlie had his first stroke on March 26, 2008. Prior to that we were an active retired couple, spending time together and also having independent activities. We went to the theater, traveled, and did a lot of things with our grandsons, including frequent sleepovers. Charlie served on four boards and found time to roller-blade and play golf and tennis. I took some art classes, played bridge, and was contemplating volunteering as a docent in a museum or as a literacy teacher at an inner-city school. I also went to the Y three mornings a week for water aerobics. Now we are at a place where both of us are living one life... his. I have learned to do all the things he took care of, in addition to my normal tasks. I have attended all his therapies with him and attempted to give him as stimulating a life as possible. Charlie has had four strokes, and each one took a little more away. He is wheelchair-bound and cannot use his right arm or leg. He had gotten some speech back and was able to say simple phrases, but the fourth stroke took that away. Fortunately, his comprehension is rather strong. This allows us to enjoy TV, movies, HD operas, theater and other activities that give us pleasure.

For several years, the Adler Center and Mona Greenfield's program provided the structure of our lives. Charlie attended Adler two days a week. It is a place where everyone has aphasia. Even though people are at different levels, there is a level playing field, such as there would be in any social club. Each person has the opportunity to pick classes of interest. There is so much laughter and happiness at the center. They also have an excellent support group for caregivers. All the caregivers are the spouses and partners of people with aphasia. We enjoy each other's company, and we have bonded very well. We found Mona's program to be a good program that emphasized academic skills, such as language, word recognition, comprehension, and reading.

In addition to the above, Charlie also received private physical therapy, occupational therapy, water therapy, and speech therapy. All of these things led to enough improvement that we decided to go to the Michigan Aphasia Center for a total immersion program. We were very pleased with the results. His level of reading improved, as did his ability to speak. We came home ecstatic about his progress.

Things continued in this way for a while, until Charlie had another stroke, which took away most of his new found skills. When Mona had to move her location and it was no longer accessible to us, we were fortunate to find excellent aphasia programs at Hunter College and Teachers College. Now, Charlie attends weekly, private speech sessions at Teachers College. The graduate students who work with him are well-supervised and excellent—patient, caring, and bright.

We were able to enroll Charlie in adaptive waterskiing, airplane gliding, and sailing. These classes were offered through both Helen Hayes and Burke's Rehabilitation Programs. He loved these wonderful opportunities for excitement and adventure.

As hard as I try to have some private time to enjoy my own interests, conflicts in the timing of Charlie's program and what could be my activities make it difficult to pick me over him. I still have been able to keep my bridge game and a once-a-month book club. My goal is to be able to get back to the Y two times a week, so I can have some physical activity. I hope to change the balance of my time spent with Charlie, so I can have time to pursue some interests of my own. My plan is to change the ratio from Charlie 95%/ Jan 5% to Charlie 65%/ Jan 35%. I hope I can succeed! I have found that our social life has changed very significantly. The people at Adler now have more significance in our lives.

CHAPTER 8

Aphasia Advocacy

Let's Make Aphasia Front Page News
Ellayne S. Ganzfried, MS, CCC-SLP

(Reprinted with permission of Ohio Speech-Language-Hearing Association (OSLHA) online journal, eHearsay.)

When was the last time you saw or heard the word aphasia in the media? It seems that a week doesn't go by when autism, breast cancer or Alzheimer's disease aren't featured in the news; Aphasia, however, is rarely discussed and often overlooked even when an opportunity may present itself. http://www.nytimes.com/2014/03/17/opinion/ when-speech-wont-come-understanding-aphasia.html Elman, Ogar, & Elman, 2000 noted "to the public and the media, aphasia is an unknown disorder." According to Elman and her colleagues (2000), aphasia is under-represented in the media, yet most people who do know about aphasia learn about it from newspapers, magazines, radio, TV and the movies (Code et al., 2010; Simmons-Mackie et al., 2002). There are almost two million people with aphasia in the U.S., yet the lack of awareness and information about aphasia is as devastating as the disorder itself. A survey done by The National Aphasia Association (1988) found that 90% of informants reported public awareness of aphasia to be minimal. International surveys of aphasia awareness were consistent with those conducted in the United States with an average of 7.34% having some knowledge of aphasia (Code et al., 2010). The consequences of limited public awareness have been well documented and include the level of funding for services and research, quality of services, reintegration into the community and workplace and psychosocial adjustment for those with aphasia and their families (Elman et al., 2000; Simmons- Mackie et al., 2002; Flynn et al., 2009)

If it is clear that awareness is needed then what can be done? What are the barriers?

Aphasia is an acquired communication disorder that impairs a person's ability to process language, but does not affect intelligence. It is an impairment of language, affecting the production or comprehension of speech and the ability to read or write (www.aphasia.org). The dictionary defines awareness as the state or condition of being aware; having knowledge; consciousness (Random House, 2014).

Issues Contributing to Decreased Awareness

There are several issues contributing to the difficulty in raising awareness of aphasia. An interesting one to consider is that aphasia is not a disease, in and of itself, but rather a symptom of disease or injury. The main causes of aphasia are stroke and brain injury and often aphasia is but one of the consequences, albeit a major one. The person and his/her family are overwhelmed by this life-changing experience and are seeking guidance for all the resulting impairments. Unfortunately, physical impairments are often prioritized, as they have greater impact on the person's discharge status and are also easily visible.

Health professionals need to be better educated regarding aphasia resources, communication strategies and long term improvements that can be made. Increased awareness and advocacy tools need to be incorporated into the assessment and intervention process at all levels of care. Mavis (2007) reported that neurologists, in collaboration with speech-language pathologists, should be in a position to develop educational programs to increase public awareness. Aphasia education should be standard in the training curriculum for all health professionals to insure better patient satisfaction and outcomes.

Another issue relates to the stigma associated with the inability to communicate preventing public understanding and acceptance of those with aphasia. Key to raising awareness is providing information yet a survey of consumers done in 2011 by Hinckley & Ganzfried rated aphasia resources as "somewhat difficult to find." (Hinckley et al., 2013) Ease of access to information is certainly a barrier to increased awareness. A critical goal is to encourage the development of community resources, advocacy strategies and support networks. People with chronic aphasia spend most of their time with family and friends, in shops, restaurants and other community activities;

They spend much less time with health care professionals or with social services (Code, 2003). The need for "wideranging and increased training and awareness-raising among the general public about communication disability" has been advocated by Cottrell (2001, p. 102). This is further support for targeting awareness activities to the public and specifically within local communities.

Additional barriers include the perception of stroke and subsequent aphasia as occurring in the elderly. The number of people aged 15 to 44 hospitalized for stroke jumped by more than one third between 1995 and 2008, say researchers from the U.S. Centers for Disease Control and Prevention (George et al., 2011). In another study, scientists combed through more than 100 studies from 1990 to 2010 studying stroke patients across the world and also used modeling techniques when there was not enough data. They found the incidence of stroke has jumped by one quarter in people aged 20 to 64 and that those patients make up almost one-third of the total number of strokes. (Feigin et al., 2014).

They add that strokes in young people have a "disproportionally large economic impact," as they can disable young patients before they reach their most productive years. In a younger person there may be the added burden of careers, relationships and raising children which will require additional resources for a longer period of time. Aphasia is experienced in 21-38% of all individuals with acute strokes (Berthier, 2005) and there are reportedly 795,000 strokes per year (www.strokeasociation. org) so you do the math. This speaks to the exceptionally high incidence of aphasia in stroke yet it is rarely addressed.

Awareness of aphasia was one of seven themes identified when looking at the environmental barriers and facilitators to community participation by people with aphasia (Howe et al., 2007) It would seem that if we aim to create "aphasia friendly" environments, we must first have greater knowledge and awareness of aphasia and the needs of those living with aphasia (Howe et al., 2004, 2007). The World Health Organization's (WHO) International Classification of Functioning, Disability and Health (ICF) (WHO, 2001) is used as a framework for identifying the specific barriers and facilitators that need to be considered when creating an aphasia-friendly environment.

Steps in Increasing Awareness

The most obvious way to raise public awareness is to use the word "aphasia" to describe aphasia. A main issue with the lack of awareness stems from people not hearing the word and understanding what it means. It is commonly reported by people with aphasia and their families that they left the hospital "never hearing the word aphasia." It seems easier to say that there is a problem with "speaking" or "understanding" rather than using the word aphasia. The persistence of this behavior will continue to undermine any awareness raising efforts. Speech-language pathologists were found to be one of the information sources in advocating publicity (Mavis, 2007). It is incumbent upon speech-language pathologists to encourage and support people with aphasia, family and friends in promoting public awareness. We also need to be empowering those with aphasia to self-advocate; they are the best "ambassadors" for aphasia.

Participation in public awareness campaigns like National Aphasia Awareness Month which is celebrated in June and contacting the media with public service announcements and human interest stories are excellent ways to raise awareness. Involving students in aphasia advocacy and helping to influence public policy and legislation are additional ways of increasing awareness. Aphasia awareness training for emergency responders and aphasia-friendly business programs can encourage engagement by all constituents. It would seem that there is benefit in having a public figure and/or celebrity as a spokesperson for the disorder. Parkinson's disease has had Michael J. Fox to assist in raising awareness. It is clear that the extent to which a public figure raises awareness is related to their willingness to be open and to publicly share their personal experience. Targeting awareness at the media offers the best hope for eradicating stigma because of its power to educate and influence public opinion

Founded in 1987, The National Aphasia Association (NAA) is a consumer-focused, nonprofit organization that promotes public education, research, rehabilitation and support services to assist people with aphasia and their families. The NAA's mission is to promote universal awareness and understanding of aphasia and provide support to all persons with aphasia, their families and caregivers. The NAA is the first and only national organization dedicated to advocating on behalf of people with aphasia. Resources include:

- Website (www.aphasia.org)
- Resource hotline (800-922-4622)
- National registry of aphasia support groups and affiliates throughout the U.S.
- The Aphasia Handbook: A Guide for Stroke and Brain Injury Survivors and Their Families
- Aphasia awareness training program for emergency responders;
- Aphasia friendly business program
- National Aphasia Awareness Month in June
- Multicultural task force
- Annual regional conferences.

There are similar consumer organizations in other countries such as Speakability in the United Kingdom, Association Internationale Aphasia (AIA) representing Several European Nations, and Australia Aphasia Association, to name a few. For the aphasia community, there is an overwhelming need for an organization which links consumer, research and professional organizations world-wide – an umbrella to drive the aphasia agenda forward. If we are to truly improve the lives of people living with aphasia – not just in one country, but also all over the world - we must find a united direction. A new organization, named Aphasia United, has been established to meet this need. Aphasia United's goals are to increase the visibility of people with aphasia, create formal global networks that connect people living with aphasia and the clinicians and researchers who support them, set a global research agenda and strengthen international research partnerships, and encourage best standards of practice in aphasia care. Aphasia United aims to serve as an international peak organization for aphasia consumer, research and professional organizations throughout the world (Hinckley et al., 2013).

Since its inception in 2011, Aphasia United has held two International Summits, established four working groups, invited advisory council members and affiliates to become involved and been endorsed by the World Stroke Organization (WSO).

Treatment for people with aphasia has evolved through time. There have been some new treatment models that have been created including the Life Participation Approach to Aphasia (LPAA, Chapey, Duchan, Elman, Garcia, Kagan, Lyon & Simmons-Mackie, 2000) and other social approaches. Unfortunately, there have been changes in our healthcare systems and insurance reimbursement which has limited the coverage for speech-language treatment. This has motivated the creation of aphasia community groups and aphasia centers which may be a cost effective way of providing the ongoing communication support needed. Unfortunately, there are not a sufficient number of aphasia centers and groups to meet the growing needs in the community. There have been several studies that have shown the value of aphasia center participation including the effectiveness of conversation treatment. (Bernstein-Ellis and Elman, 1999; Elman, 2007, 2010; Simmons-Mackie et al., 2010) Technology has become a new avenue of exploration for aphasia treatment and has allowed people with aphasia to work on skills independently and for a longer period of time.

A significant advance has been the understanding that a person's speech can continue to improve for years after acquiring aphasia; there is no plateau. The principles of experience-dependent neural plasticity have inspired different treatment approaches and research. We now know that the damaged brain "relearns" lost behavior in response to rehabilitation (Kleim & Jones 2008). Research is being done in a variety of areas and has included looking at intensity of aphasia treatment, i.e., Constraint Induced Language Treatment (CILT); dosage i.e., Intensive Comprehensive Aphasia Programs (ICAP); other ways of treating aphasia i.e., using computer technology, pharmacology/medications such as memantine (Namenda) and piracetam, and/or directly impacting the brain to enhance the effects of the speech and language therapy through electrical or magnetic stimulation of the cortex. Future directions need to include additional support for evidence based practice, innovation and determining alternative treatment delivery models in our changing health care system. Of course this is all closely tied to our ability to increase awareness of aphasia and the understanding that it is a chronic condition that impacts individuals throughout their lifetime.

We are definitely moving in the right direction and have had notable accomplishments, including Congress proclaiming June as National Aphasia Awareness Month; however, there is more work to be done. There is compelling evidence that international public awareness campaigns and advocacy initiatives are critical to increasing recognition and understanding of aphasia which will directly impact the quality of life for people with aphasia. It is only through the coordinated efforts of all constituencies that we can move the aphasia agenda forward and make a difference on the world stage. Let's look for the day when aphasia is front page news!

Aphasia Training for First Responders
Stephen Symbolik, MA

Communication is crucial in emergency situations, but aphasia can affect an individual's ability to state his or her name or understand a firefighter saying, "Follow me." Stressful situations often exacerbate the effects of aphasia—people may have even greater difficulties expressing themselves or understanding what others are saying. Many stroke and brain injury survivors are already at risk in crisis situations because of their physical impairments; those with aphasia as well can be rendered almost completely vulnerable.

While emergency service personnel, such as EMTs and firefighters, rarely receive training on aphasia, they are in fact more likely to encounter a person with aphasia (PWA) than someone with multiple sclerosis, cerebral palsy, or muscular dystrophy (Will & Peters, 2004). However, many of these first responders do not know what aphasia is, much less how to communicate with a person with the disorder. Unfortunately, because few emergency responders are specifically trained to deal with people with aphasia, they may mistake the disorder for mental illness or other conditions. This can lead to misunderstandings that make efforts to help people with aphasia useless or even dangerous. The pioneer training project recounted here arose out of one such situation.

With seed funding from the Christopher and Dana Reeve Foundation in 2008, the National Aphasia Association (NAA) created a pilot project to train first responders in the New York metropolitan area. The project objectives were to educate police, firefighters, and EMTs in New Jersey, New York, and Connecticut about aphasia, so that they could recognize, communicate with, and respond more effectively to people with aphasia in routine encounters or in emergency situations. Specifically, the NAA was trying to educate police, firefighters, and EMTs so that they would recognize the signs of aphasia when interacting with the public. In addition to becoming familiar with aphasia and its different forms, our goal was also to have first responders recognize the Aphasia Awareness symbol/sticker (Figure 1), which is now being used by PWAs on their vehicles and homes.

Several outlines for training were developed for this program, taking into account differing audiences, time allotments, and depths of interest. For example, training outlines for EMT's who have medical training were developed to include more specific information regarding the physiological types of aphasia, whereas training for police and firefighters concentrated more on identification and communication techniques. All training modules delivered both started and ended with the Aphasia Quiz (www.aphasia.org), so that we could measure the effectiveness of our short training courses. Evaluation forms were used to determine satisfaction and knowledge gained from the training, as well as to obtain data for research relating to community needs.

The various PowerPoint training presentations were combined into a training package, which included an informational brochure, the Aphasia Awareness symbol/sticker, copies of the Aphasia Identification Card (figure 2) and the Aphasia Education for Emergency Personnel DVD, developed in 2008 by the Aphasia Advocacy Foundation of New Hampshire and the University of New Hampshire.

The NAA met and exceeded its target goals for the pilot project. 450 trainers for the New York City Police Department (NYPD) were trained in aphasia awareness. They, in turn, were charged with bringing this training to approximately 25,000 police officers and personnel. The NYPD has incorporated the training into a permanent lesson plan in their command-level training program. Training was delivered to 25 chiefs of Middlesex County, New Jersey fire department. A relationship for ongoing training was established with the Nassau County (NY) Police Training Academy, which delivers all training to police, firefighters, and EMTs in the county. Training was also conducted in Fairfield County Connecticut. Training for EMTs and EMS providers then expanded, and we conducted training for Northwell Health (previously North Shore-LIJ Health System) Center for EMS. In January 2010, the Law Enforcement Training Directors Association of New York State (LETDANYS) invited us to provide training at its conference in Albany. The word "aphasia" was getting out there. The value and relevance of this training was recognized and took off, especially with police, EMTs and EMS workers. It turns out that the best catalyst for training is word-of-mouth endorsements, even if those words don't come easily!

Beyond education about aphasia, the training focused on strategies to better communicate with PWAs, including explanations and demonstrations of several very simple communication techniques. A PWA can usually answer questions with a simple yes or no, a thumbs-up or thumbs-down, pointing to the words "yes" or "no," or even a nod of the head up or down. Trainees were asked to think about the way in which they asked questions: Were their questions open-ended or closed? Obviously, open-ended questions are much more difficult for a PWA to answer, because these questions require the respondent to search for words. Using closed questions allows the respondent to answer simply affirmatively or negatively. Thus, instead of an officer asking, "Where do you live?" he or she could ask, "Do you live at the address on your driver's license?" The latter makes more sense and is easier for the PWA to answer with a yes or no, a gesture, a thumbs-up, or a nod. No doubt there are emergency situations in which it is not possible to wait for a response, however, it is imperative that the PWA is given time to speak or answer as best as they can when possible.

Initially, we encountered some roadblocks and delays to training. Most of the barriers to our objectives had their genesis in the fact that targeted audiences were unfamiliar with aphasia and were, therefore, hesitant to follow-up on requests to deliver training. These roadblocks were expected and served to both highlight and document the very reason that aphasia awareness training for emergency responders was needed. It was very likely that people with aphasia were not being recognized, served, identified, or treated appropriately in emergency situations. The opportunity for aphasia training was featured on the NAA website, in community presentations, and in other media. This facilitated the opportunity for PWAs, speech-language pathologists, caregivers, students, and professors to make inquiries about the training program and materials.

As the training programs expanded, people with aphasia wanted to help train the targeted communities. Incorporation of personal experience and perspective was encouraged, adding a new dimension to the training. It also served to empower the PWA to advocate for him or herself and assisted with his or her rehabilitation. A perfect example of this was when Avi Golden, a paramedic who suffered a stroke, became an integral part of the training team. Because of his contacts in the EMT/EMS world, we were able to train hundreds of emergency responders in New York, New Jersey, and across the country. Emergency responders connected with him professionally and used their newly learned communication strategies to interact with him in real time. The training became real, and its applicability to professional skill sets became clear.

An exciting collaboration occurred with Dr. Michael Cassara, Associate Program Director in Emergency Medicine with Hofstra Northwell School of Medicine (previously Hofstra University North Shore-LIJ Health System). Through his efforts, we were able to train incoming students and residents in Emergency Medicine. Our training performance objectives were successfully incorporated into the teaching methods for both first-year medical students and residents learning patient communication techniques. The first training incorporated PWAs into clinical demonstrations, requiring the students to attempt diagnosing aphasia in a simulated emergency situation. The second training reviewed the overall objectives of training with residents, reminding them that good communication is a key component in a fruitful patient-doctor interaction. Further discussions have focused on using this training as a model for other medical schools throughout the country.

As we continued to focus on and provide training to emergency responders in the tri-state area, the number of volunteers wanting to train emergency responders outside this region continued to grow. Hundreds of volunteers were trained to use the training materials, which were easily adaptable to specific audiences. Not surprisingly, and despite the often unbridled enthusiasm of the volunteers, they too found that initiating training was not an easy task. Persistence, however, paid off, and we began to see the emergence of a national training program.

In Chicago, Patricia LaMontagna, began training emergency personnel in aphasia awareness. Patricia was a retired police officer from the Cook County Sheriff's Police Department, who had suffered a stroke in 2009 that resulted in aphasia. She had remarkable success with the training program, not only in Chicago, but also in canvassing the entire state of Illinois. Patricia simply would not take no for an answer to a request for training. In 2014, she received the Inspire Award from Presence Resurrection Medical Center, which "recognized her for her tireless efforts in supporting and educating stroke survivors, their families, and caregivers," including hundreds of aphasia awareness trainings.

It is worth a moment to point out that, without exception, the aphasia training was entirely orchestrated through volunteers. Men and women offered their time freely to bring awareness to the cause of aphasia. We also had strong interest from students studying speech-language pathology, nursing, and related disciplines. There were student trainers from many states including New York, Pennsylvania, Florida, North Carolina and Texas. In January 2014, we were invited to provide training for the first freshman class of students who were becoming EMS-certified with Associate's Degrees at Kingsborough Community College in Brooklyn, N.Y.

These students weren't afraid of rejection and had the savvy to use innovative technology to capture targeted audiences. Many caregivers also became aphasia training advocates and conducted training with PWAs as part of their rehabilitative process.

Rodney Wolfe, a caregiver for his wife who has aphasia, is a construction inspector with the City of Allen Engineering Department in Allen, Texas. He devoted countless hours to training people about aphasia in remote and rural areas of Texas. He was also one of the first volunteers to conduct training via webinar in July 2011. This was entirely new ground for him, and he exemplifies the type of volunteers that were dedicated to aphasia awareness. Because of volunteers like him, training began to take place not only in unexpected places, but also in some of the most remote parts of the country.

We have found that these training programs impart simple and easily understood material that not only increases the professionalism and effectiveness of first responders, but also contributes to the overall safety and well-being of PWAs. This is precisely because police, fire, and emergency personnel that have participated are now equipped to respond and communicate effectively with those with aphasia.

What started out as a program specifically focused on first responders began to achieve a more global audience. Inquiries began to pour in from other interested parties who saw the value of having their employees trained in aphasia awareness. These included hospitals, schools, banks, restaurants, and retirement communities. The training program is adaptable to differing audiences including hospitals, schools, banks, restaurants, and retirement communities. An alliance was formed with the Snyder Center for Aphasia Life Enhancement (SCALE) in Baltimore, Maryland. In January 2011, the center launched a campaign targeting businesses with the goal "to educate local businesses about aphasia and advocate for the rights of people with aphasia to receive access to their products and services." Business owners were invited to participate in a free opportunity to increase their business by better serving people with aphasia. (More information about this particular program can be obtained by visiting them at scalebaltimore.org.)

An aphasia-friendly business training program was created by working collaboratively with some of SCALE's training models. In Baltimore, SCALE had the advantage of working with small, local businesses that saw the economic advantages of understanding how to cater to PWAs. These businesses were able to better serve the very people who were receiving services from SCALE. In other states, the business structure was markedly different. It was difficult to be successful on a large, corporate level, so efforts were focused more upon local businesses. What could have easily been win-win couplings, were instead often-missed opportunities. This, however, failed to deter us and we persevered, casting the training net to include a wider audience.

An encounter in 2012 with a woman who served in the vestry of an Episcopal Church in Manhattan led to training at this parish. This resulted in some local media exposure, and, shortly thereafter, we also conducted training at several synagogues in Manhattan. These trainings served as models to other trainers, who also conducted aphasia awareness training in other churches, temples, and congregations around the country. It was not missed that the major faiths in the United States, each being people whose faith was grounded in the "Word," were in fact, fertile ground to train and teach people about those who can no longer use, or have difficulty in using, words to communicate. I am hopeful that religious communities will continue to be the voice of the voiceless, and that aphasia awareness training in some small way has played a part in this endeavor.

Beauty and cosmetology schools were also targeted. It seemed like a good fit, considering that people with aphasia still get their hair cut and use beauty services offered by this multi-million dollar industry. In July 2012, Therese Vogel, owner of Tiffin Beauty Academy in Tiffin, Ohio, had her entire staff and student body trained in aphasia awareness. The Hair Design Institute in Manhattan also trained staff and students in aphasia awareness. The advantages of understanding aphasia and how to communicate to persons with aphasia was not lost on them. Many realized that they could cultivate a loyal clientele by utilizing the communication techniques taught during training. Aphasia awareness training dovetailed nicely with communication skills that were already included in the curriculums of most cosmetology schools. In 2013, an article on the training program was published in Beauty Link magazine, the publication of the American Association of Cosmetology Schools (AACS).

Retirement homes and communities also requested training. Some, after hearing about our training program, realized that they had persons with aphasia living in their facilities, yet staff had never explained to other residents what aphasia is or how to communicate to the people with aphasia. We welcomed these opportunities to share the skills required for mutual communication.

Final Thoughts on Training

From the small seed-money obtained from the Dana and Christopher Reeve Foundation, which was originally used to provide for pilot trainings in New York, New Jersey, and Connecticut, aphasia awareness training for both first responders and for businesses expanded into 32 states. The force and momentum of this training was all driven by dedicated volunteers and persons with aphasia. Training materials were also shared with people in Australia, Canada, Great Britain, Mexico, Peru, New Zealand, and South Africa. No doubt that with additional funding these training programs could become global in scope and implementation. The addiction for instant communication ushered in by technology also brings the blessing of easy dissemination of information. On a shoe-string budget, it was possible to connect hundreds of people and give them a new way to think about words and communication. Many of the techniques used, such as speaking slowly, being more articulate, watching body-language, and making eye contact during conversation are very effective ways for anyone to improve their language and interactive people skills. Being mindful and paying attention to what someone is saying or trying to say also has a boomerang effect. As you become more present to others, they become more present to you, and lines of communication are opened, ushering in real opportunities for dialogue, compromise, and understanding to occur.

Trying to understand someone else's reality, such as a person with aphasia, presents a challenge to discard many of the assumptions, often erroneous, we have about language, words, and how we tend to judge people on their ability to use words. Universally, the essence of each of us resides in that right side of the brain. When the left side of the brain is damaged and the result is aphasia, we don't disappear or go away. We can be every bit as present to ourselves as we were before the brain injury. New studies and dynamic discoveries about the brain have been emerging in the scientific community. Studies have shown that the brain is very plastic. In many instances, it is possible for PWAs to recover language skills. Talking, communicating, and interacting or being given the opportunity to interact is exercise for the brain. The more a person with aphasia practices, the better the chances for some type of recovery. It is hoped that these modest training goals that were shared with so many, by so many, continue to bear fruit in our communities. Keep using your words, but remember, they don't define who you are; they are simply the symbols and vehicles in service that you choose to express your true self!

Figure 1

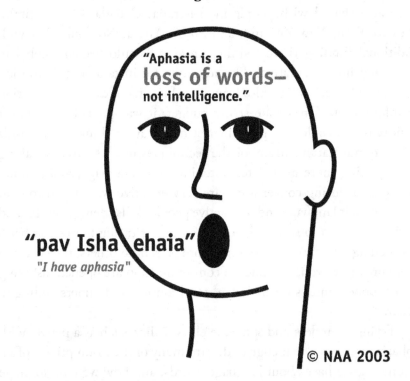

Aphasia Awareness Sticker

Figure 2

Name: ————————————————————————
Address: ————————————————————————
Phone: ————————————————————————
Emergency Contact: ————————————————
Phone: ————————————————————————
For more information about living with aphasia, contact:
National Aphasia Association
350 Seventh Avenue, Suite 902
New York, NY 10001
1-800-922-4622 / www.aphasia.org
This card was made possible by an award to the Rehabilitation Institute of
Chicago from the National Institute on Disability and Rehabilitation Research,
U.S. Dept. of Education, Washington, D.C. (Grant no. H133B031127)

Please Take Time To Communicate

I have aphasia (uh fay'zhuh)
a communication impairment.

My intelligence is intact.
I am not drunk or
mentally unstable.

Aphasia ID Card

EPILOGUE

The Voice of Aphasia

Rebecca K. (Rivky) Herman, MS, CCC-SLP

Speech-language pathologists frequently envision a career through which they hope to be able to touch the lives of their clients. They quickly discover that in fact their clients are often the greatest and most touching influence on their lives. The following illustrates such an experience:

In a dimly lit room we sit opposite one another separated by only a rickety wooden desk
Yet, we are miles apart
He sits frightened on an island far from home
Each tear that falls from his swollen eyes descends into the ocean surrounding the quiet and desolate place
Miles of salt water surround him
He struggles to call for help, to communicate just one thought
Yet, he cannot find the words; he can only cry
He yearns for someone to hear his weakened voice
In response, he hears only the echo of his voice
His voice is the voice of aphasia

His spirit acts as a wave traveling up to the heavens and down to the depths
It is raised up with every achievement
It flows down with each setback
Yet, as waves of tears crash fiercely into the shore, he gathers great strength
He dives in to rescue others who are drowning as they fight to escape
The waves begin to dance in the darkness; his spirit dances along
Cha cha to the heavens, two steps on the ground
Soon others on the island join in with the dance
A circle of hope is formed
His strength is the strength of a hero

As those on the mainland study the depths of the sea
As they explore that which lies deep within the tears
They see someone in the distance dancing the tango on salty waters
He soon rises above the waters as he choreographs a new piece
A once hopeless man with a weakened voice transforms into a leading dancer
He educates those around him regarding those trapped on the island
He saves others from drowning and teaches them how to dance
His cries turn to song as he creates awareness to those far and wide
The circle of hope grows larger as others sing and dance along
His lessons are the lessons of a great teacher

He no longer hears only the echo of his voice
I hear his song as I long to guide him home
Each session brings him closer to the mainland
Each lap he swims
Each word he speaks
Each sentence understood
Each cha cha to the heavens
Each note perfected
Each thought communicated
His story is the story of a survivor

He reminds those on the mainland to appreciate gifts which are too often taken for granted
While studying, three pages may appear too difficult for some to learn
For others, three words are too difficult to speak
Some can tell their friends and family that they love them
Others can love, but cannot express their love in words
Some can name their dreams for the future
Others can dream, but cannot say their own name
Some can sing
Others can only cry
His voice is the voice that awakens

Moving Forward: Lessons Learned
Mona Greenfield, PhD, LCSW, CCC-SLP

Many survivors are part of our story. Each voice of the person with aphasia (PWA) and caregiver is courageous, unique, and precious. These are real people who struggle with aphasia or with a loved one with aphasia. It is through this very humane dynamic that we share an understanding of the whole person—not just a diagnosis.

To make this journey successful, we remain open to the extraordinary potential and hope that our participants put forth. We remain spirited, believing in the changes we see each day. When days are difficult, we continue to support our participants and believe that we learn from each day. Whole healing and the "new normal" guide us on this journey. To survive means to accept that life has changed, but there is still potential for growth, progress, fulfillment, and success.

Stories live on and unfold. These real stories are just some of a tapestry of lives and hopes from persons with aphasia.

Aphasia is a label. Persons with aphasia are much more than a communication impairment. Even though communication affects a person's ability to express, emote, comprehend and share in social language contexts, there are many ways for persons with aphasia to continue to engage in the world. The most important thing is for them to continue to search and develop whatever creative and alternative methods allow them to move forward.

We have been so privileged to have received and shared in these stories, learning and growing as professionals as we look to understand the island of aphasia from multiple perspectives and experiences. My team continues to believe in achievable goals in living life and finding happiness by accepting the "new normal".

So what have we learned?

Lesson 1: Never Give Up!
After a stroke or brain injury, individuals are often told that there is a finite recovery and rehabilitation window, but there is always hope; as speech-language pathologists, we never stop working, living, and believing.

One of my participants, Fran, told a story about a long walk that made her very tired. She took small steps, went slowly, and little by little she completed it and was proud. She realized that the rehabilitation process takes time. She has been working with me for ten years now and continues to practice and develop her skills. Through ongoing supports and social and cognitive stimulation she feels encouraged and continues to be hopeful. Throughout her emotional journey and rehabilitation, we have approached Fran as a person not just with a diagnosis of aphasia, but from a holistic perspective, an integrative approach connecting mind and body that nurtures the healing process and allows for successful growth.

Lesson 2: Re-energize!

It is important for therapists to keep striving for the best and most functional therapy for their participants. Some days are more successful than others, as persons with aphasia and those involved with their care are constantly confronting new challenges. Each day is a chance to move forward in some way, whether in the rehabilitation of skills or in working to accept the "new normal." Factors such as fatigue, stress, and depression all affect the total functioning of a PWA. It helps both the therapist and participant to rest and breathe, calming and re-energizing the mind and body.

Lesson 3: Always Seek Alternatives

Most often when faced with obstacles resulting from aphasia, there are other ways to communicate and resume life. Communication alternatives range from low-tech to high-tech, including gesturing, forming letters with hands and fingers, using alphabet boards, paper and pencil, and iPads. If there is a desire to communicate, there is a way to facilitate it. If one of these alternatives is frustrating, try a different approach. The PWA appreciates connecting in a meaningful and social way—with respect and belief that he or she can both continue to partake in successful communication and be valued as a conversational partner in a satisfying relationship.

Various adaptations can also be made for activities in a daily routine and even for a possible return to work. In all cases, a lower stress environment with a slower pace can certainly help PWAs feel more comfortable. Mobility assists, such as walkers, wheelchairs (simple or motorized), and local transportation for individuals with disabilities, offer options for PWAs to participate more fully and independently in community life.

Lesson 4: Stay in the Moment
Planning is necessary, but it is most important to focus on the now and allow whatever emotion comes to be accepted. If emotions and feelings are overwhelming, counseling support can help. Once emotions are felt and shared, the process of letting go can begin. There are many days when the person with aphasia may feel broken. These feelings need to be addressed and the individual needs to be supported as he or she goes through the healing process.

During these times, it can help for those with aphasia to make lists of what currently brings them hope and joy, and then incorporate these items into their daily activities. They can also use positive affirmations to create more fulfilling positive emotions and feelings. Affirmations can be listened to or spoken to reinforce increased self-esteem and potential for healing.

Lesson 5: Do Not Be So Hard on Yourself!
PWAs tend to compare their present functionality to how they were prior to having aphasia. While having high self-expectations for recovery can be a great motivator, being self-critical and focusing on life prior to aphasia, though quite normal, is counterproductive with regard to recovery. It is important to accept what is and strive toward better days and increased self-confidence. Support is needed to help the person with aphasia realize that communication may not necessarily improve as quickly as one would like; however, even small positive changes need to be addressed and appreciated. It is a long journey and it helps to gain an understanding of what his or her new normal is.

Lesson 6: Caregivers Count!
All of those people who are integrally involved in helping the person with aphasia need to be supported and included in therapy and plans

for his or her recovery. Within this ecosystemic framework, which integrates medical, social, and psychological rehabilitation into one cohesive process, the PWA cannot heal without the love and care of those in their world. Therefore, caregivers must be supported, informed, and included in a mutual contract with the PWA to facilitate maximal progress.

It is through the many voices in this book that we have learned about the journey with aphasia. Rehabilitation means understanding, supporting, and respecting the whole person. To effectively treat aphasia one must utilize a compound bio-psycho-social approach and work to build a ecosystemic understanding of the person—their aspirations, their struggles, and their will to continue life.

In a personal email to me, Al shared these words:

> *Thank you for making it easier for us by having groups after our hardships! It was 3 years in September I joined, & I remember how scared I was! Remember me crying? Laughing is so much better. In the PA group I see the "newbies" & their caretakers, how scared & frightened they are & us old-timers tell them we walked before where they are now, but they are not alone! Don't ever be afraid to ask for help!*

GLOSSARY

Acalculia
The loss or impairment of math/number skills.
www.dictionary.com/browse/acalculia

Agraphia
The loss or impairment of normally acquired writing skills.
www.dictionary.com/browse/agraphia

Alexia
The loss of previously acquired reading skills due to recent brain damage.
www.dictionary.com/browse/alexia

Anomia
A condition characterized by difficulty retrieving words; individuals with anomia often use circumlocution (wordy and indirect language) to express an idea when unable to retrieve the desired word or words.
www.asha.org/Glossary/Anomia/

Apraxia (of speech)
A motor speech disorder. The messages from the brain to the mouth are disrupted, and the person cannot move his or her lips or tongue to the right place to say sounds correctly, even though the muscles are not weak. The severity of apraxia depends on the nature of the brain damage. Apraxia can occur in conjunction with _dysarthria_ (muscle weakness affecting speech production) or _aphasia_ (language difficulties related to neurological damage). Apraxia of speech is also known as _acquired apraxia of speech_, _verbal apraxia_, and _dyspraxia_.
http://www.asha.org/public/speech/disorders/ApraxiaAdults/

Cognition

The mental action or process of acquiring knowledge and understanding through thought, experience, and the senses.
www.oxforddictionaries.com/definition/english/cognition

DSM 5

Diagnostic and Statistical Manual of Mental Disorders (DSM) is the standard classification of mental disorders used by mental health professionals in the United States and contains a listing of diagnostic criteria for every psychiatric disorder recognized by the U.S. healthcare system.
http://www.dsm5.org/Pages/Default.aspx

Dysarthria

A motor speech disorder. It results from impaired movement of the muscles used for speech production, including the lips, tongue, vocal folds, and/or diaphragm. The type and severity of dysarthria depend on which area of the nervous system is affected.
http://www.asha.org/public/speech/disorders/dysarthria/

Emotional Lability

Excessive emotional reactivity associated with frequent changes or swings in emotions and mood.
https://books.google.com/books?isbn=0803639090

Expressive Language

The use of words, sentences, gestures and writing to convey meaning and messages to others. www.childdevelopment.com.au/sound-awareness/65

Fine Motor Skills

The coordination of muscles, bones, and nerves to produce small, precise movements.
https://medlineplus.gov/ency/article/002364.htm

Gross Motor Skills

The coordination of muscle, bones and nerves to produce large, general movements.
https://medlineplus.gov/ency/article/002368.htm

Hemiparesis
A muscular weakness or partial paralysis restricted to one side of the body.
https://books.google.com/books?isbn=0877799148

Human Resources Administration or Department of Social Services (HRA/DSS)
The department of the government of New York City in charge of the majority of the city's social services programs. HRA helps New Yorkers in need through a variety of services that promote employment and personal responsibility, while providing temporary assistance and work supports. Its regulations are compiled in Title 68 of the New York City Rules. HRA is the largest city social services agency in the United States. It has a budget of $9.7 billion, employs over 14,000 people, and serves over 3 million New Yorkers.
https://en.wikipedia.org/wiki/New_York_City_Human_Resources_Administration

Melodic Intonation Therapy (MIT)
One of the few accepted treatments for severe, nonfluent aphasia is Melodic Intonation Therapy (MIT), a treatment that uses the musical elements of speech (melody & rhythm) to improve expressive language by capitalizing on preserved function (singing) and engaging language-capable regions in the undamaged right hemisphere. Melodic intonation therapy is facilitated by a specially trained clinician, such as a speech pathologist.

Norton, A., Zipse, L., Marchina, S., & Schlaug, G. (2009). Melodic Intonation Therapy: Shared Insights on How it is Done and Why it Might Help. *Annals of the New York Academy of Sciences, 1169*, 431–436.
http://doi.org/10.1111/j.1749-6632.2009.04859.x

Neuroplasticity
The ability of the nervous system to respond to intrinsic or extrinsic stimuli by reorganizing its structure, function and connections.

Cramer, S. C., Sur, M., Dobkin, B. H., O'Brien, C., Sanger, T. D., Trojanowski, J. Q., ... Vinogradov, S. (2011). Harnessing neuroplasticity for clinical applications. *Brain, 134*(6), 1591–1609.
http://doi.org/10.1093/brain/awr039

Perseveration

In psychology and psychiatry, perseveration is the repetition of a particular response, such as a word, phrase, or gesture, despite the absence or cessation of a stimulus, usually caused by brain injury or other organic disorder. In general English, perseveration (vb: "to perseverate") refers to insistent or redundant repetition, not necessarily in a clinical context.
https://en.wikipedia.org/wiki/Perseveration

Semantic Feature Analysis (SFA)

A therapeutic technique that is used for the treatment of naming deficits occurring with aphasia. SFA is used to guide the patient in identifying important semantic features of the target word. This approach is believed to help activate the semantic network that surrounds the target word to aid in its retrieval.
https://communicationtherapyforadults.wordpress.com/2014/03/01/semantic-feature-analysis-sfa/

Propofol

Marketed as Diprivan, Propofol is a short-acting, intravenously-administered, hypnotic/amnestic agent. Its uses include the induction and maintenance of general anesthesia, sedation for mechanically ventilated adults, and procedural sedation. Propofol has been referred to as milk of amnesia (a play on words of milk of magnesia), because of the milk-like appearance of its intravenous preparation.
https://en.wikipedia.org/wiki/Propofol

Traumatic Brain Injury (TBI)

Traumatic brain injury, also known as intracranial injury, occurs when an external force traumatically injures the brain. TBI can be classified based on severity, mechanism or other features. Head injury usually refers to TBI, but is a broader category because it can involve damage to structures other than the brain, such as the scalp and skull.
https://en.wikipedia.org/wiki/Traumatic_brain_injury

BIBLIOGRAPHY

American Stroke Association. (2014) Impact of stroke (Stroke statistics). Retrieved from http://www.strokeassociation.org/ STROKEORG/AboutStroke/Impact-of-Stroke-Stroke-statistics_UCM_310728_Article.jsp

Awareness. (n.d.). Dictionary.com Unabridged. Retrieved July 14, 2014, from Dictionary.com website: http://dictionary.reference.com/ browse/awareness

Bernstein-Ellis, E. & Elman, R.J. (1999). The efficacy of group communication treatment in adults with chronic aphasia. *Journal of Speech, Language, and Hearing Research*, 42, 411-419.

Berthier, M. L. (2005). Poststroke aphasia: Epidemiology, pathophysiology and treatment. *Drugs and Aging*, 22, 163–182.

Bright, F. A. S., Kayes, N. M., McCann, N. M., & McPherson, K. M. (2013). Hope in people with aphasia. Aphasiology, 27(1), 41-58.

Castka, Karen and Abbanat, Ginette and Holland, Audrey and Szabo, Gretchen

Potential benefits of participating in an aphasia theater program. In Clinical Aphasiology Conference: * Clinical Aphasiology Conference (2009: 39th: Keystone, CO: May 26-30, 2009) /: (2009). http://aphasiology. pitt.edu/archive/00001972/

Cherney, L. R., Oehring, A. K., Whipple, K., & Rubenstein, T. (2011). "Waiting on the Words": Procedures and outcomes of a drama class for individuals with aphasia. Seminars in Speech and Lang, 32, 229-242.

Code, C., Simmons-Mackie, N., Armstrong, E., Stiegler, L., Armstrong, J., Bushby, E., Carew-Price, P., Curtis, H., Haynes, P., McLeod, E., Muhleisen, V., Neate, J., Nikolas, A., Rolfe, D., Rubly, C., Simpson, R. & Webber, A. (2001) The public awareness of aphasia: an international survey. *International Journal of Language and Communication Disorders*. 36 (Suppl.), 1-6.

Code, C. (2003) The quantity of life for people with chronic aphasia. *Neuropsychological Rehabilitation*, 13, 379-390.

Code, C. et al, (2010). International Comparisons of the Public Awareness of Aphasia. Presentation at 14th International Aphasia Rehabilitation Conference, Montreal.

Cottrell, S. (2001) How do lay people perceive individuals who have communication disabilities, and in particular, aphasia? — Unpublished dissertation submitted in partial fulfilment of the MSc in Clinical Communication Studies, Department of Language and Communication Science, City University, London.

Croteau, C., Le Dorze, G., Marchoux-Fortier, M., & Getty, M. (2008, June). What effects does the participation in a theatre workshop have on individuals affected by aphasia? Poster session presented at the 13th International Aphasia Rehabilitation Conference, Ljubljana, Slovenia.

Davidson, B., Worrall, L., & Hickson, L. (2008). Exploring the interactional dimension of social communication: A collective case study of older people with aphasia. Aphasiology, 22(3), 235-257.

Davis, G.A. (1983). *A survey of adult aphasia*. Englewood Cliffs: Prentice Hall.

Davis, G. A. (2007). *Aphasiology: Disorders and Clinical Practice* (pp. 33-39). Boston, MA: Allyn & Bacon. Adapted with permission. Retrieved from http://www.aphasia.org/aphasia-definitions/

Elman, R., Ogar, J., & Elman, S. (2000). Aphasia: Awareness, advocacy, and activism. *Aphasiology*, 14, 455–459.

Elman, R.J. (2007a). *Group treatment of neurogenic communication disorders: The expert clinician's approach.* Second edition. San Diego: Plural Publishing.

Elman, R.J. (2007b). The importance of aphasia group treatment for rebuilding community and health. *Topics in Language Disorders*, 27(4), 300-308.

Feigin, V. L. et al. Global and regional burden of stroke during 1990–2010: findings from the Global Burden of Disease Study 2010. Lancet 383, 245–255 (2014).

Fromm, D., Holland, A., Armstrong, E., Forbes, M., Mac Whinney, B., Risko,A., Mattison, N. (2011). "Better But No Cigar": Persons with Aphasia Speak about their Speech. Aphasiology, 25(11): 1431–1447

Flynn, L. Cumberland, A., & Marshall, J. (2009). Public knowledge about aphasia: A survey with comparative data. *Aphasiology*, 23, 393-401.

Ganzfried, E., & Hinckley, J., The persistent needs of people living with aphasia: Results of a national survey. Clinical Aphasiology Conference, North America, June 2012. http://cac.library.pitt.edu/ocs/index.php/cac/cac2012/paper/view/261

Ganzfried, Ellayne S. (2014). When speech won't come: understanding aphasia. *The New York Times*. Retrieved from http://www.nytimes.com/2014/03/17/opinion/when-speech-wont-come-understanding-aphasia.html

George, M.G. et al. (2011). Trends in stroke hospitalizations and risk factors in children and young adults: 1995-2008, *Annals of Neurology*. doi:10.1002/ana.22539 or http://doi.wiley.com/10.1002/ana.22539.

Hardy, B. (1978). Narrative as a primary act of mind. In M. Meek, A. Warlow & G. Barton (Eds.) The cool web.New York: Atheneum.

Hilari, K., Needle, J. J., & Harrison, K. L. (2012). What are the important factors in health-related quality of life for people with aphasia? A systematic review. *Archives of Physical Medicine and Rehabilitation*, 93(1 Suppl), S86-95. doi: 10.1016/j.apmr.2011.05.028

Hinckley J. Finding messages in bottles: Successful living with aphasia as revealed by personal narrative. Topics in Stroke Rehabilitation. 2006; 13:63–67. [PubMed: 16581631]

Hinckley, J. J. (2008). *Narrative-based practice in speech-language pathology: Stories of a clinical life.* San Diego: Plural Publishing.

Hinckley, J. J., Hasselkus, A., & Ganzfried, E. (2013). What people with aphasia think about availability of aphasia resources. American Journal of Speech-Language Pathology, 22, S310-S317.

Hinckley, J., Worrall, L., Ganzfried, E., & Simmons-Mackie, N. (2013). World beat: A united international voice for aphasia. *The ASHA Leader*, Vol. 18, 34-35.

Hobson, M. R. (2006). The collaboration of music therapy and speech-language pathology in the treatment of neurogenic communication disorders: Part I on diagnosis, therapist roles, and rationale for music. *Music Therapy Perspectives*, 24(2), 58-65.

Howe, T., Davidson, B., Worrall, L., Hersh, D., Ferguson, A., Sherratt, S., & Gilbert, J. (2012). 'You needed to rehab families as well': family members' own goals for aphasia rehabilitation. International Journal of Language & Communication Disorders, 47(5). doi: 10.1111/j.1460-6984.2012.00159

Howe, T., Worrall, L., & Hickson, L. (2004). What is an aphasia-friendly environment?
Aphasiology, 18(11), 1015-1037.

Howe, T., Worrall, & L., Hickson, L. (2008). Interviews with people with aphasia: Environmental factors that influence their community participation. *Aphasiology*, 22 (10), 1092-1120.

Kleim, J.E., & Jones, T.A., (2008) Principles of experience-dependent neural plasticity: implications for rehabilitation after brain damage. *Journal of Speech, Language, and Hearing Research*, 51 (1), S225-S339.

Landy, R. J. (1994). *Drama therapy: Concepts, theories, and practices* (2nd ed.) Springfield, IL: Charles C. Thomas.

Levin, T., Scott, B.M., Borders, B., Hart, K., Lee, J., & Decanini, A. (2007). Aphasia talks: Photography as a means of communication, self-expression, and empowerment in persons and aphasia. *Topics in Stroke Rehabilitation*, 14(1), 72-84.

LPAA Project Group (2000). Life participation approach to aphasia: A statement of values for the future. ASHA Leader, 5(3), 4-6. <www.asha.org/public/speech/disorders/LPAA.htm>. Reprinted in R. Chapey (2008). (Ed.). Language intervention strategies in aphasia and related neurogenic communication disorders. (5th Ed.). Baltimore: Lippincott, Williams & Wilkins.

Mavis, I. (2007). Perspectives on public awareness of stroke and aphasia among Turkish patients in a neurology unit. *Clinical Linguistics & Phonetics*, 21, 55.

Mesulam, M.M. (1982). Slowly Progressive Aphasia without Dementia. *Annals of Neurology*, 11, 592-598.

Mesulam, M.M. (2001). Primary Progressive Aphasia. *Annals of Neurology*, 49:425-432.

Moreno, J. L. (1985). *The autobiography of J. L. Moreno, M.D. (Abridged)*. Boston: Moreno Archives, Harvard University

National Aphasia Association. (1988). Impact of aphasia on patients and families: Results of a needs survey. Unpublished report. Retrieved from http://www.aphasia.org/

Peterson, C. (2006). Art therapy. In E. R. Mackenzie & B. Rakel (Eds.), *Complementary and alternative medicine for older adults: A guide to holistic approaches to healthy aging* (pp. 111-134). New York: Springer.

Rao, P.R. (1995). Drawing conclusions on the efficacy of 'drawing' as a treatment option for patients with severe aphasia. *Journal of Aphasiology,* (9), 59.

National Institutes of Health, National Institute of Neurological Disorders and Stroke. (1999). Stroke: Hope through research. Retrieved from www.ninds.nig.gov

National Stroke Association. (2003). National Stroke Association's complete guide to stroke. Retrieved from www.stroke.org

Shadden, B., & Hagstrom, F. (2007). The role of narrative in the Life Participation Approach to aphasia. Topics in Language Disorders, 27(4), 324-338.

Simmons-Mackie, N., Code, C., Armstrong, E., Stiegler, L. & Elman, R. (2002). What is aphasia? Results of an international survey. *Aphasiology,* 16, 837-848.

Simmons-Mackie, Raymer, A., Armstrong, E., Holland, A. & Cherney, L. (2010). Communication partner training in Aphasia: A systematic review. *Archives of Physical Medicine and Rehabilitation,* vol. 91, 1814-1837.

Sparks, R.W., Holland, A.L. (1976). Melodic intonation therapy for aphasia. *Journal of Speech and Hearing Disorders,* (41), 298-300.

UK Connect. (2015). Living with aphasia. Retrieved from http://www. ukconnect.org/impacts-and-effects-of-aphasia.aspx

Ward-Lonergan, J., & Nicholas, M. (1995). Drawing to communicate: A case report of an adult with global aphasia. *International Journal of Language and Communication Disorders,* 30(4), 425-491.

Will, M. & Peters, J. (2004). Law enforcement response to persons with aphasia. The Police Chief, December 2004, 20-24.

World Health Organization (WHO). (2011). *World Report on Disability.* Retrieved from www.who.int

Worrall, L., Sherratt, S., Rogers, P., Howe, T., Hersh, D., Ferguson, A., & Davidson, B. (2011). What people with aphasia want: Their goals according to the ICF. *Aphasiology,* 25(3), 309-322. doi: 10.1080/02687038.2010.508530

Printed in the United States
By Bookmasters